THE GREENWICH WEIGHT LOSS AND DIABETES DIET

Christopher J. Mosunic,
PhD, MBA, RD, CDE
&
R.D. Martin

Contributors

Erica Christ, MS, RD, CDE
&
Chef Gavin Pritchard, RD

ISBN Number: 1480027588
ISBN-13 Number: 9781470027589

Library of Congress Control Number: 2012918465
CreateSpace Independent Publishing Platform
North Charleston, South Carolina

ACKNOWLEDGEMENTS

Special thanks to Katie Meskell; Bernard "Bud" Barton; Karen Jurgens; Sue Colmant; Sara Paulson; Michael Howerton; Joshua Hrabosky, PsyD; Steward McCalley, M.D.; Anthony Alleva, M.D.; and to those individuals who prefer anonymity because there is still a stigma attached to labels such as "obese" or "diabetic". Each unselfishly contributed in their own way, and each of their contributions is greatly appreciated.

THE GREENWICH WEIGHT LOSS AND DIABETES DIET

Chapter 1

THE FIRST STEP IS THE HARDEST

This self-help book is for those of us with type 2 diabetes who want to lose weight, keep it off, and don't want to be miserable just for the sake of being thinner. Written by a decreasingly overweight person with diabetes, it is based on the work of one of the foremost experts in the field of diabetes and weight loss. More accurately, this book is a "rewritten" version of an unpublished manuscript and treatment principles developed by Chris Mosunic, PhD, a clinical psychologist and registered dietitian who specializes in diabetes and weight loss. I'll explain this unusual collaboration between this clinician and his patient, me, shortly. However, don't fret; this book is not about my personal journey other than to explain how this got started.

It is hard to come to the realization that you want help to lose weight, but it's even harder to ask for help. Most people with diabetes who desire to lose weight don't look for help from a book, so this makes you a bit different than most…in a good way, of course. You believe in yourself and want to make changes in your life. Unfortunately, not everyone does. Many of us approach weight loss with what we believe is common sense: we try to watch our diet, cut back on sweets, carbs, or calories, exercise a bit more, and hope for the best each time we step on the scale. Many of us will approach our "diet" with great expectation and we feel strongly committed—so much so, we religiously restart it every Monday morning after it falls apart sometime during the prior week! Perhaps a few of us will even try some snappy herbal remedy that promises to melt our fat like dripping candle wax. Surely, we've all tried diets that required we deny our hunger through superhuman willpower—something we quickly learned we can't live with on a permanent basis. No wonder they're called crash diets…we crash! It is hard enough for non-diabetics to lose weight, and having diabetes only makes our endeavor more complex. Unfortunately, in most cases, the above approaches are the only ways we know how to lose weight. We now have a much better option, one that not only works for both our weight and our diabetes, but is also comfortable and rewarding enough to sustain our success in a simple, continuous, lifetime achievement. We'll call it *The Greenwich Diet*, but it is not a diet in the usual sense of the term. It is all about learning why we eat and controlling the forces that compel us to overeat. It is about finding greater satisfaction, not learning how to live with deprivation.

Deep down, most of us believe that our inability to lose weight is our own fault: we lack willpower, or we have some unspeakable character weakness. Many of us cringe at the thought of doctors' appointments, knowing they will probably direct their attention to our weight regardless of their specialty. Often, our doctors and other professionals will scare us repeatedly by detailing the medical consequences of our condition—as if we aren't already painfully aware of them. Health professionals are usually "ill-equipped" to motivate us, and they find their scare tactics actually work sometimes, at least in the short-run. Hey, that's why they use them! More than a few of us have dropped a few pounds because of pressure or fear of embarrassment if we don't lose weight. However, as you've probably discovered, negative pressure only works for a short while. After our mandatory medical lecture, we often get angry and go on a diet to show our doctor that we can lose weight. After we demonstrate our success at the next doctor's visit, some of us even stop for a fast food fix on our way home to congratulate ourselves. Shall we have a show of hands please?

It is difficult to be overweight and have diabetes, and many of us believe it is so extremely difficult to lose weight that we've decided to just learn to live with our situation. Some of us call it "self-acceptance". Others label it "resignation". Those of us with "abundant" weight have had our share of humiliating moments and have stories we share only with our closest friends…if anyone at all. No doubt you've noticed our problem with excess weight, although common, has a stigma attached. We are judged and treated differently, but never in a nicer way. Sometimes, even the professionals we turn to for help have negative attitudes towards us because of our excess weight. It is uncomfortable, humiliating and even depressing to know we are the targets of anti-obesity campaigns and held responsible for contributing to spiraling healthcare costs. Knowing this, it is hard to hold our heads up high, and it is all too easy to turn to food for comfort. Eating immediately helps us forget our problems and feel better. What a vicious cycle this is! Of course, not all of us have put on enough weight to feel this stigma. Those of us who are taking action early on and our weight becomes a serious problem deserve a hearty congratulations!

You will come to learn your weight problem has nothing to do with character weakness or lack of willpower. Instead, it has to do with some tricky but correctible biochemistry and patterns of living and thinking that can be changed without having to stand on your head or rely upon unrealistic willpower. When you finish this book, please lend it to someone you know whom has lost faith in their ability to lose weight. This book is written for them too—it is just that it is very hard to get them to grab a copy without first wrestling them to the ground.

Getting started on something new is often the hardest part. Although the story of how a book gets started is usually part of a preface, many readers skip prefaces, so the story is included here. You'll see why.

I was facing other medical issues which were made more serious because of my abundant weight, so I "agreed" to see Dr. Mosunic only because I didn't have the gall to say "no" to my doctor who made the recommendation. I hold him in very high regard, and I was worried he would think less of me if I refused his recommendation to seek help. I dutifully faked a cooperative demeanor and agreed to go my hospital's diabetes and weight loss center where he referred me, but only so I could say I tried it and it didn't work. My major concern was how long I'd have to put up with a darn regimented weight loss program before I could justifiably call it a failure. I had parts of my rejection speech already prepared. It was persuasive, one of my best, and I was sure I could save face with my referring doctor. Within a couple of weeks after I called the diabetes and weight loss clinic, I finally had my first appointment. Oh joy.

I fully expected some arrogant, fit person to tell me to eat less, or worse, ask me to monitor my food intake—perhaps even in writing! I was told earlier that Dr. Mosunic would ask to be called Chris—another cheap trick, I figured. I spent my career in human services, and met all types. I felt prepared. I knew the ploy. However, I was immediately relieved when I met Chris, because I realized I had the bulk to toss him across the room if provoked! As it turned out, I didn't have to engage in any form of self-defense that day. Actually, my self-protective instincts never reemerged after we shook hands and started talking. He talked "with" me, not "at" me. I wondered if he was really a fat man trapped in a thin man's body. Ironically, I was later to learn I wasn't that far off; he was fat in his preteens, a terrible age to be fat. I know that from personal experience. It also appears he is predisposed to diabetes and has to watch his diet carefully.

I felt physically lighter after my first meeting. I did have a strange feeling, however; it might have been a slight touch of optimism, but I figured that odd and unfamiliar sensation would eventually pass. I wondered if he realized he met one of the potentially most resistant patients in his career. Then again, maybe we all feel this lousy about our weight, and all share as deep a desire to protect ourselves. I only know how I feel about my own weight problem, and I'm acutely aware of how others react to my size. I hate it. I always figured my weight problem was my personal issue, different from others. It turns out I'm not that unique after all. You probably aren't either.

I surprise myself by admitting to Chris that I worry I have an obsessive disorder. I explain I have an uncontrollable, constant hunger, and the thoughts of food and eating keep popping into my mind regardless of what I'm doing. I even dream of food! I watch the "hoarder" programs on TV, and wonder if I am hoarding food in my stomach—if I am an "internal hoarder"! I am totally taken by Chris's response...no, actually "stunned" by it. He, no doubt, heard this complaint before. He assures me, with total confidence I know is genuine, that I do not have an obsessive disorder. He explains the constant thoughts and hunger I have are due to the biochemistry involved in diabetes and a reaction to the foods I eat. He assures me it can be corrected (which it later is). He asks what kind of commitment I am willing to make. The best and most honest response I can come up with is "fair"—I'll give it a "fair" shot I tell him. I add that I would be more invested if I see results. He didn't flinch at my masked challenge.

Chris offers to let me read a book he wrote that was still awaiting publication. His book explains the biochemistry as well as many other things related to diabetes that can contribute to weight gain. I find he doesn't leave any stone unturned: he explains the biochemistry of hunger and eating; what to eat to control hunger; how our food environment tempts us to eat; how some of us eat to help us deal with emotions and negative moods; exercise; and food preparation, etc. He not only explains all these things, but gives practical advice: a way out of my mess, an escape hatch. I eventually find his book of such great value because of my own eventual success, that I ask him if he'd be willing to let me reshape his book and ideas into a self-help book. I explain that most of us who want to lose weight and manage our diabetes do not have access to a specialty clinic such as his, and because of this, many of us are at a great disadvantage. He agrees, and is open to having me rework his approach into a self-help, format. I didn't realize at the time that he is one of if not *the* foremost authority on weight loss for people with diabetes. If I had known this before asking for an okay to transform his book, I might have been a bit more reluctant to make the request.

This book's sole purpose is to help people like us—including those of us who might have to be cajoled into reading this book (which is not to say you are one of them). The credit for the concepts, ideas, and recommendations are Chris's and the other professional contributors. This book is re-sculpted from his manuscript. I am taking advantage of the opportunity to use my own style and voice, and speak directly to you as a fellow patient and diabetic. A hidden agenda (I guess I'm coming clean now) is to also influence some of the professionals who happen upon this book. It might help them appreciate our problem from a patient's perspective. Certainly, not all professionals require sensitivity training, and certainly not those professionals who have taken the time to read this book. If you are one of these outstanding individuals, please consider giving this book to a peer you know whom might benefit from a little sensitivity training. You know who they are! If you fear they'll be insulted, simply sign someone else's name to a belated birthday card and attach it to the book. It works every time. However, if you received this book with a belated birthday card attached, you may have reason for concern.

Having a professional clinician and their patient co-author a book is highly unusual. Although one of us provides the ideas and the other provides the expression, you'll hear both voices as one. The guiding philosophy behind this person-centered perspective and approach to this book is summed up by a wonderful quote from Richard David Bach, who says, "You teach best what you most need to learn." Both authors find this to be true (but would substitute the word "need" for "want"). You'll find out why later.

Although this book is written for people with type 2 diabetes, it is also a fantastic weight loss solution for those who don't have diabetes. It is not intended for people with type 1 diabetes. Whether you are looking for a way to maintain your current body weight, shed a few pounds, or you are one of us who wants to cut our body weight in half, this approach will work for you. Because it is hard to lose substantial weight without turning parts of your life around (or alternatively stated, turning your life around sometimes requires losing substantial weight), this book is as much about creating a meaningful and enjoyable life as it is about shedding pounds. Food and eating permeates every aspect of our lives, so it is simply impossible to deal with food and eating in isolation. You'll soon discover that overeating, in many cases, is just the visible part of the iceberg, and if you don't pay attention to what's below the surface, you may not reach your destination. *The Greenwich Diet* recommends not only a healthy way of eating to achieve weight loss and better control of diabetes, but it also recommends a healthy way of thinking so we rely less upon food for comfort and satisfaction.

The solution to weight loss is neither simple nor quick. Sorry. This approach to weight loss is for those of us who have come to learn the hard way that magical weight loss approaches don't work after the initial (although often impressive) weight loss. Losing weight and keeping it off is not just about what to eat and when to eat. True success is about improving your life, adding to your happiness, and trading up for a more satisfying life that relies less upon food for emotional sustenance.

To accomplish this weight loss and lifestyle transformation, you'll want to learn a few new things about food and eating, and you will shortly be invited to look at your eating and your life differently. You'll also want to invest a reasonable amount of time and effort. The most important thing is that although it requires effort and willpower, it requires neither unreasonable effort nor superhuman willpower. You'll be able to live with this new approach to eating. You'll be thinner and happier than you are now. If you are already happy, you'll be happy *and* thinner! The solution to our weight problem is about increasing satisfaction in life, not lessening it. You will not be expected to feel deprived, miserable or constantly hungry. *The Greenwich Diet* is a solid, non-gimmicky, medically proven approach that puts together all the things that influence our eating so we can attack the problem from all angles: (1) the biological urge to overeat, (2) the psychological reasons why we eat, and (3) our food environment that constantly tempts us to eat. This approach is not about giving up the pleasure and satisfaction; it is instead about trading up to a better way of living. It is as much about gaining pleasure as it is about losing pounds. That's why it works.

"You" throughout the book means you, the reader who is overweight and who has diabetes. "We" and "our" refers to those of us who have diabetes and who are overweight; it does not refer to the authors. Medical, psychological and other professional jargon is avoided as much as possible. "Diet" usually means the foods we eat as omnivores and not a short-term eating plan unless it is obviously meant as such. Labels such as "obese" or "morbidly obese" are avoided, unless they emphasize a point or refer to a medical diagnosis. "Fat" is used freely. It is assumed you have a basic understanding of diabetes, because basics are not covered in this book. If you want a good introduction to diabetes or if your information is out of date (yes this happens), you are highly encouraged to check with your healthcare provider or track down a certified diabetes educator (CDE).

You'll come to understand how your biology, psychology and environment all influence your eating and how to work with each of them to overcome the obstacles you face trying to lose weight. You'll learn about what foods to eat and in what combinations to eat them in order to control your blood sugar levels and tame a ravenous appetite. You'll find food preparation tips and discover great recipes; learn how to increase your motivation; discover how to break through any resistance you have towards exercise; and finally, meet others like yourself who sought help, lost weight, and improved the quality of their lives. Most of all you'll learn how to be both thinner *and* happier—a win-win solution.

A good place to start on your goal to lose weight and take better control of your diabetes is to understand the nature of hunger and why we eat. What you'll learn may amaze you. Hunger is not a subject many of us have thought much about; we're either hungry or we're not, and when we're hungry we eat. Right? Well…

✲ ✲ ✲

Chapter 2

WHAT REALLY MAKES US EAT?

We need to eat to survive. We know that. We also know that the excess weight we carry is because we take in more fuel in the form of food than we use. The extra fuel we consume gets stored as fat for later use. Unfortunately, we don't seem to get around to using up our abundant fat reserve—well, at least those of us who are overweight.

Fat storage helped our cave-dwelling ancestors survive periods when food was sparse. Actually, up until 200 years ago or so, humans typically went through cycles of "feasts" and "famines". There were times when food was plentiful and times when it was not. Those ancestors who were more successful at overriding our built in biological "slow down" or "stop eating" mechanism, and who were therefore able to store up lots of extra energy in the form of body fat, survived the lean times better than their thinner, non-fat-storing neighbors. This is known as the "thrifty gene hypothesis". If you want, you can toy with your friends by saying you have the "thrifty gene syndrome" (even though there is really no such diagnosis). Those ancestors able to pack on extra pounds were able to celebrate their survival by engaging in intimate activities that passed on the genes responsible for their superior ability to store fat. This process of favoring weight-gainers over non-weight-gainers went on for many generations. The majority of people today have ancestors who were expert at putting on body fat and overriding the satiety signals. You are one among many.

Although our bodies are stuck in modes more useful in the past than now, we are living in a world very different than our ancestors. Although it may not have been very thoughtful of our ancient forbearers to pass down those fat-storing genes, we have to give them credit for leaving some incredible cave paintings, many of which appear to be rather tasty looking animals. Do you think the cave paintings were really a menu where you point at your selection and someone runs out and hunts for it?

We eat for many reasons other than to keep our body properly fueled. Understanding why we eat is much more complex than most people think. If we really want to lose weight and manage our diabetes, we'll have to understand all the different reasons why we eat. Understanding all the reasons is not as challenging as it sounds. The more you learn, the easier it will be for you to lose weight. Also, as you continue to read, there is a good chance you will find much of what you learn both surprising and interesting. You may even have a few "ah-ha" moments. Really.

The general belief is that people are overweight because they lack willpower. Lack of willpower is not the cause of excess weight gain or the inability to lose weight. Oddly, even after we learn this, many of us overweight people still tenaciously hold on to this misconception; we think it probably applies to others…but not us. We can, and do, back up our belief with a rap sheet of our failures. We convince ourselves, that at least in *our* particular case, lack of willpower is really the deep down, secret cause of our excessive weight. Sadly, this erroneous belief can discourage many of us from seeking help for fear we'll be exposed and called out for our "character fault". We become discouraged. The last thing we want is another failure under our belt. To add to the problem, we all know that if someone is convinced they'll fail, they will fail. So why would we even want to try? Many of us have walked that walk—or, more accurately, gangplank.

This is not to say you can lose weight and manage your diabetes without any willpower whatsoever. We'll leave those lofty claims to the snake oil sellers—those offering effortless, quick fixes. Losing weight will take effort, but the effort will be well within your ability. You will not be expected to live in a constant state of hunger or end your meal before you are satisfied. You'll soon discover why you were unsuccessful in the past, and realize it was not due to your lack of willpower. This discovery is very reassuring and encouraging.

Give yourself credit for trying to find solid help. You are obviously open to learning a new approach or you wouldn't have turned enough pages to make it this far. Even if you stole or borrowed this book, at least you are reading it. Not everyone takes this important step. Understandably, many of us are simply too afraid to learn more about our problem. We don't want to discover that we ourselves are the problem. One thing to warn you about upfront is to be vigilant… very, very vigilant…against that old "lack of willpower" tape. Don't take it out of storage and allow it to replay in your head again if you encounter challenges along the way. If it enters your mind, just think of it as just your fat protesting out of self-protection. Soon, you'll have a whole new perspective on your weight problem, and you'll have the tools to lose weight and better manage your diabetes.

There are various reasons why we *decide* to eat or not eat. Notice the use of the word *"decide"*…hmmm…are we onto something here? Most of us are familiar with the mental ping-pong game we play: "Mmm, a cookie (burger, pizza, goat, etc)! No, I shouldn't eat that cookie. I don't need that cookie. We'll, I'm in a lousy mood, and I haven't eaten that much today anyway, so why shouldn't I? I deserve a break, I deserve a reward, and eating it will make me feel better. I deserve to feel better…" You know how the internal ping pong dialogue usually ends with… "Chomp, chomp, chomp, yummmmm!" If you are now tempted to jump up and grab a sweet, you know how powerful even simple cues can be…and boy, we're certainly surrounded by them!

The problem is that we can't win the ping-pong match consistently, and we eventually become defeated. We blame ourselves for giving in, and tell ourselves we lack willpower. However, if our eating problem is as simple as mastering this simple internal dialogue, being overweight wouldn't be so widespread, and you wouldn't be reading this book. Sure, our rational mind plays an important role, but it is only one of many influences that determine why we decide to eat or not. Our thought process, mood, physiology, lifestyle and food environment all play a role. Here are some reasons why we eat:

1. Because we talk ourselves into it.
2. Because we're bored.
3. Because we're sad or stressed.
4. Because we're happy and/or celebrating.
5. Because others want us to eat.

6. Because our physiology tells us to eat (using complex signaling pathways).
7. Simply because the food is there!

Yet, more important than all of the above reasons why we eat is that we eat because we've given up hope that we can do anything to change the self-destructive path we are on. Think about how often you've thrown in the towel. Although it is not our conscious intent to self-destruct, the end result of throwing in the towel often is, sadly, self-destructive. Failed attempts to lose weight provide us with even more proof we can't change, and we simply give up hope. It is a vicious cycle. It is extremely important to realize there are reasons why we "give in"…and it is not for lack of willpower. You will soon discover the reasons we "give in".

In addition to eating to survive physically, we also eat to survive mentally. Overeating serves a purpose in the short run—or at least tries to serve a purpose: it helps us (or appears to help us) maintain some kind of mental balance in this teeter totter world. The problem is that the balance isn't working properly. The consequences can be annoying to some and devastating to others. Diabetes adds an additional malfunction (and challenge) to our balancing act, and for many of us, our struggle with weight is literally a life and death struggle.

This struggle has given rise to the unattractive labels "obesity," or worse, "morbid obesity". At least to many of us, "obesity" is our forbidden "O" word. The label usually makes us cringe; it makes our skin crawl. To many, the term is repulsive, disrespectful and even worse than being called childish names. Don't forget, however, that the terms "obesity" and "morbid obesity" are formal medical diagnoses, so we're going to hear those terms whether we like them or not. Actually, we are becoming quite accustomed to those terms. They are now used so frequently in the media during the last few years that they don't have the sting they once had. We can agree to use those unattractive or diagnostic labels here amongst ourselves, if we agree that, when used, they are not meant to be demeaning or a put down. Instead, we can use those powerful labels to remind ourselves of the harsh reality many of us face. Just remember, if those words seem to jump off the page to slap or provoke you; they are used to remind us we are in hot water and may have a serious health condition.

Food is like a drug. We need it, crave it, can't go without it, and we like the way it feels when we ingest it. Our body needs food to function. It provides the energy needed to complete the tasks of everyday living. Therefore, we cannot "opt-out" of eating in order to cure what is often called the "obesity/diabetes epidemic". Further, our inability to "opt out" explains why addiction treatment approaches often fall short in treating serious weight problems and diabetes. You can go "cold turkey" with alcohol, smoking, or drugs, but you cannot give up food.

We eat for many different reasons, and if you toss all the reasons in the air, you will find they land, more or less, into three different categories:

1. Physiological: Our body chemistry has various ways to compel us to eat.
2. Social: We are surrounded by food, people enjoying food, and what seems to be a constant barrage of cues to eat. We'll call this our "food environment".
3. Psychological: We eat in an attempt (albeit a short-sighted attempt) to maintain psychological balance.

To be successful, we'll want to understand and deal with all three. Now, the above three groups are not neat little piles; they overlap and influence each other, and at times even join forces. Think of them as different pieces of a jigsaw puzzle, but keep in mind that the mind and body are not two separate entities.

✻   ✻   ✻

Chapter 3

HELP! WHAT'S MAKING ME SO HUNGRY?

You are surrounded! A number of nefarious forces are working in collusion to get you to eat…no, overeat! They are ruthless and belong to one of three factions: the "Biochemistry Bombardiers," the "Environmental Encouragers," or the "Psychological Persuaders". Although separate entities, they send secret messages back and forth and team up against you often. Your only defense against them is to understand them and maneuver your way around them. But, before you figure how to outsmart and disarm them, you'll first want to understand how they work. Although later chapters will explain the practical measures you can take to thwart their efforts to make you eat more than you need, you'll first want to discover how each of the three factions works. Here's the inside scoop:

Biochemical Signals of Hunger, Eating and Weight Gain

For many people struggling to lose weight, especially for people with diabetes, understanding how the physiological aspects of hunger work is nothing less than amazing—and oddly reassuring. You'll discover that you confuse, at least in some situations, biochemistry with willpower.

Many things are happening on a physiological level to control hunger, eating and weight. We are bombarded by biochemical signals telling us when to eat, when not to eat, when to store energy, and when to release stored energy. Worse, when eating we release dopamine, a chemical associated with addiction! Now, don't let the idea of learning a little biochemistry scare you. It is more interesting than academic and there is a good chance that a few little light bulbs will to go off in your head as you read. Others might notice the glow.

Your body ensures you eat food on a consistent basis by delivering signals to your brain to eat. It doesn't matter how big or small you are. Hunger and blood sugar are two important signals that compel us to eat. You'll also discover how dopamine affects us. If you associate dopamine with drugs, you are correct.

HUNGER AND BLOOD SUGAR: TWO IMPORTANT SIGNALS TO EAT

When the bladder of an animal fills, a signal is sent to a lower part of the brain containing two important components (the basal ganglia and the hypothalamus if you are particularly interested). The signal to the lower brain tells animals to empty their bladder. If the animal is a bear in the woods, for example, it doesn't think twice about it, and the bear "waters" the nearest tree. Humans on the other hand, and some well-trained cats and dogs, use the very same circuitry of the lower brain to learn to *not* act on the urge to urinate, despite the urge being a very strong one. The same area of the brain responsible for telling an animal to "go" is the same part telling it to "stop". The same lower brain responsible for primitive functions such as urinating is also responsible for eating! When our stomach empties, the lower brain sends us signals to eat—much like the lower brain sends signals to urinate. Consequently, the urge to eat when the stomach is empty is equivalent to the urge to urinate when the bladder is full. Surprising, isn't it?

Now, let's apply this to willpower. If your bladder is full, how long will you last before giving in? Perhaps a few minutes will go by, or maybe even an hour or two at the most. If you can distract yourself, perhaps you can last a bit longer. However, your urge will become stronger over time, and soon it will be hard to think of anything else other than your urge to urinate. When you are able to finally urinate, it will be one of the most pleasurable experiences you can have. The same is true of the urge to eat when the stomach is empty. Perhaps you'll last a few minutes or even an hour or two with an empty stomach, but you'll eventually succumb to the urge to eat. When you do give in, it will be tremendously pleasurable—so pleasurable in fact, that it is likely to result in binge eating.

DOPAMINE

To add insult to injury, the brain will reward you for fulfilling the urge to eat by releasing the neurotransmitter dopamine. Dopamine shooting around your brain makes you feel great! So great, in fact, that it is often associated with drugs such as cocaine and amphetamines. It is also thought to be part of the reward system of the brain! Notice the first two letters of dopamine: "do". When dopamine is released we want to "do" it again. It feels so good, we lose track of our long-term goals and focus on getting more dopamine. We can get more dopamine simply by eating more. In most circumstances, food is usually only a few steps or arm lengths away. It's also cheap, comes in many shapes, flavors, and sizes and is looking for us as hard as we are looking for it! The bottom line is the urge to eat is just too primal and strong to fight, and the substance we're after is readily available. When we add dopamine to the other biochemical events going on, we're outmatched! Incidentally, this also explains why breakfast skippers are likely to be those with the greatest weight. The longer you go without eating, the greater is your urge to eat. Further, a greater amount of dopamine will be released when you finally do give in. Consequently, your binge will be even larger, as if your efforts to "go without" food are being punished. The first step in losing weight and controlling diabetes is to stop this binge eating cycle.

UNDERSTANDING DIABETES AND WEIGHT LOSS

Type 2 diabetes is a metabolic disease characterized by high blood sugar levels (glucose) in our blood. The high blood sugar is because we've developed a resistance to the insulin our pancreas produces, or in some cases, also because we do not produce enough insulin. Insulin removes excess sugar from our blood.

If you have diabetes or pre-diabetes, losing weight is more difficult. That's because of the "blood sugar rollercoaster" which greatly alters our hunger and eating patterns. A person without diabetes has a blood sugar range of roughly 80 to 120 mg/dl (milligrams per deciliter) in their bloodstream at any time. When they approach 80, they are more likely to feel hungry, and when they approach 120, are more likely to feel full. Those of us with diabetes have a much wider range, and consequently, much wider hunger cues. A diabetic's blood sugar may go down to 50 mg/dl (the blood glucose level you determine with the standard test strip), whereas a non-diabetic will not. For a diabetic, a 50 mg/dl blood sugar level is a "wild card," meaning that the results are unpredictable. It may result in extremely ravenous hunger, or it may result in nausea. If it does result in a ferocious appetite, the brain will be telling us to eat decadent (sugary and fatty) foods to bring our blood sugar level back up. We then eat a tremendous amount of food, that consumption brings our blood sugar up to a level much higher than a non-diabetic's. The unfortunate part is that we diabetics will not feel full until our blood sugar is very high. This is one reason why we often overeat. As our blood sugar starts to soar, our body releases more insulin, a hormone that brings blood sugar levels down. Too often, we produce too much insulin and our blood sugar falls precipitously. The low blood sugar then signals decadent eating once again, and we go back up the rollercoaster's incline. This "ride" sometimes continues all day. The net result is weight gain. Apparently, you wandered on this ride when the attendant was distracted, and now don't know how to get off. You might even be tightly strapped in.

Our diabetic blood sugar rollercoaster is *in addition* to the normal hunger cues that non-diabetics have. So, it's much tougher for those of us with diabetes to lose weight than someone without diabetes. Further, our brain runs primarily on blood sugar (glucose), and when our blood sugar becomes low, our brain becomes a very unhappy and demanding organ. Because our brain controls our body, if it is able to muster the strength, it will signal the body to consume large amounts of sugary and fatty food to refuel itself. If, due to our diabetes, our blood sugar is low, our brain may not be able to muster the necessary strength. Consequently, it will run inefficiently, and make the low blood sugar urge to eat occur inconsistently. If this does occur, however, watch out! The combination of having a low blood sugar level and an empty stomach and trying not to overeat is equivalent to drinking two liters of water and trying not to urinate. Good luck! Fortunately, there are ways to avoid these problems.

So how do we avoid this "urge" problem? We do it by not letting ourselves get too hungry and by not allowing our blood sugar to get too low. If our blood sugar level goes low and we're hungry, we're very likely to overeat delectable foods (e.g., pizza) in copious amounts (e.g., the whole pizza). This bingeing brings our blood sugar up quickly, which our brain may greatly appreciate for a few minutes. Shortly after, however, our brain regrets this, because it despises blood sugars that are too high. Our brain can be quite finicky.

When our blood sugar level goes too high, our pancreas produces insulin. Insulin is a hormone that goes into the blood stream and quickly moves the sugar from the blood into the cells of the body. If we're not physically active, odds are that a great deal of that insulin will grab sugar, as well as other components of the food we eat such as fat and protein, and store them in fat cells—either in existing fat cells, making them bigger, or in new fat cells. The good news is the blood sugar is out of our bloodstream. High levels of sugar in our bloodstream will cause a great deal of damage to your veins, arteries and organs. This is why diabetes is such a harmful disease. The bad news, however, is twofold: insulin stores away most of what we eat in the form of fat, *and* our blood sugar comes crashing down.

Welcome back to the rollercoaster, because once our blood sugar goes down, the selfish, finicky brain wants to increase it again! Therefore, signals are sent to get us to eat those delectable foods again, and this puts us back up the rollercoaster. Once more, insulin is produced and fat cells are made. Our blood sugar level again goes down and the cycle goes on indefinitely. Many of us have been on this rollercoaster for decades. Fortunately, there are ways to get off the rollercoaster and again plant our feet on solid ground.

If the above brew of obnoxious biochemistry isn't enough, there is yet another piece of chemistry that might make it even harder for us heavy people to lose weight. It appears, at least in animal studies, that insulin also affects our brain's reward circuitry. If we build up a resistance to insulin due to being overweight, and we are a diabetic or pre-diabetic, we produce even more insulin. This makes it harder for us to resist food! Because eating is part of our brain's reward system, you can see why this is a problem—hey, we love rewards; they are…well…very rewarding! Insulin resistance compels us to eat more than those without insulin resistance. This too can become a vicious cycle that only gets worse as we become more resistant to insulin. Add this maddening cycle to the rollercoaster described earlier and you are on one ugly out of control carnival ride! It's enough to make you sick!

Don't worry if you feel you're a bit over your head at the moment. This isn't the easiest information to comprehend—at least initially. In time, however, you'll get it. It is worth the investment of time and energy to learn this biochemistry "stuff," because as long as you have diabetes and try to lose weight, this wacky biochemistry will be influencing your eating and affecting your health.

There is a big difference between understanding something while we read it and remembering what we read well enough to recall that information at will. One test of your ability to recall your biochemistry lesson is to ask yourself if you could explain it to someone else. Better yet, give it a real try; explain it out loud! If you do this while on public transportation, you will find people will give you extra space and you'll have lots of extra elbow room. So go ahead! If you can't summarize the above lesson in biochemistry, or find your mind doing somersaults, you are not alone…actually; you're probably in the majority. Understanding what is happening in your body regarding hunger, eating, and weight gain is extremely important. This biochemistry explanation is probably the most complicated part of this book, so don't get discouraged. The payoff for understanding this can be measured in pounds…your pounds. If you are annoyed because you are not being let off the hook, or are totally miffed by the mere suggestion you might have to reread something, or if you simply want to check the accuracy or completeness of your recall, you might find this quick review helpful:

- Our brain signals us to eat.
- The signals to eat and to stop eating come from the part of the brain that also controls our bladder (such a lovely thought).
- The signal to eat is exceedingly strong, like the need to empty your bladder.
- If you're exceptionally hungry, eating is an extremely pleasurable experience—so much so that you are primed to turn your eating into bingeing.
- Dopamine, the feel good hormone, is released when eating.
- The longer you go without eating, the greater the amount of dopamine is released, and subsequently, the greater the binge eating episode.
- Diabetics have a wider range of blood sugar levels than people without diabetes, thus more urges to eat.
- Our body tries to control the amount of sugar in our blood by releasing insulin when our blood sugar levels are too high,

and *sometimes* by releasing sugar if our blood sugar levels are too low.

- The body's ability to balance blood sugar levels doesn't work as well as it should in diabetics.
- High blood sugar levels harm our body.
- Excess sugar is pulled from the blood and stored as fat.
- An additional process whereby increased insulin is released because of insulin resistance might be involved in our brain's reward system, and this too encourages us to eat.

You know, you can review this summary again if you want; no one's watching! You'll also find pieces of the above information repeated often enough later on. So don't worry if you feel like your comprehension is less than stellar.

Here's a real kick in the pants you might have noticed: if the above biochemistry wasn't explained to you in the past, you've expected yourself to run this obstacle course blindfolded, relying upon willpower to guide you. It wasn't fair. But this is just the beginning; this is only the biochemical aspect of understanding why we eat, what we eat, and when we eat! Just be aware the biochemistry of hunger and eating is more complex than the signals just covered, but what you've learned is enough to get you off the blood sugar rollercoaster and help you to lose weight. In case you are biting at the bit to learn more about biochemical signals, see: leptin, ghrelin, GLP-1, and CCK. How do we apply this new information about hunger and eating signals in our quest to lose weight? We'll get to that after we learn more about why we eat so much of the vast array of foods available to us.

Our Surroundings Tempt Us to Eat

Although we now understand some of the major biological signals involved in eating, and we know the importance of monitoring our food intake, we also know eating doesn't happen in a vacuum. We live in an environment that surrounds us with food from every corner of this delicious planet. Foods compete for being the most delectable and accessible. Food is imbedded in the fabric of our families, our relationships, and even our culture. We often know more about a culture's food than its other social customs or history. Our environment encourages us to eat with cues that beckon us to indulge in a vast array of delectable edibles. Food even has its own TV channel in the US! We'll want to understand and control our food environment if we are to lose weight.

Every human has a default setting when it comes to eating. That default setting is to eat whenever possible. Thanks to the "thrifty genes" we inherited, we are programmed to feast in case we encounter a famine in the unpredictable future. If food is around, we are likely to eat it. Food is big business, and some of the best minds are devoted to finding ways to encourage us to eat their products. It sometimes looks as if we are living in a food-based economy. Perhaps we are.

We're inundated with environmental cues to eat. It feels, at times, like we are living in the middle of an all-you-can-eat smorgasbord. We're inundated with cues to eat when we surf the web, watch television, drive our car, or, heaven forbid, go to the mall. Each step we take we're bombarded with messages to eat. The problem is we can always eat, food is almost always available, and we don't have to go out of our way for it. Worse, it often comes to us! Humans can eat almost non-stop and we can manufacture insulin to store away every last morsel we consume. Although many of us are fighting back against big business such as fast food chains that entice us to eat delectable foods, it is fair to say the bombardment of cues is here to stay. We can complain all we want, but at the end of the day, we'll still have to learn strategies to lose weight in a food rich environment.

Humans communicate with food to convey friendship, affiliation, and warmth. "Breaking bread" has both a cultural as well as spiritual meaning. It is even used to create just the right atmosphere to conduct business meetings. The type of food served at business meetings plays an important role of setting just the right mood and promoting the agenda, hidden or otherwise. Food is the gift that every human being enjoys at some level because every human needs to eat in order to live. In fact, when greeting someone, some cultures don't ask, "How are you?" Instead, they ask, "Have you eaten?" For most of us, there is always plenty of food in our environment to eat, and our body's default setting is to eat it. We know we will enjoy every bite, even if we are stuffed to the gills.

Food relaxes us and we can sometimes feel the relaxation response kick in while we chew, not to mention relishing the dopamine flooding our brains! In the short-term, this is as good as pleasure gets. Of course we now know that we will convert this excess food into body fat and, in the long run, harm ourselves. Unfortunately, the primitive brain isn't programmed to think that way, so we have to outsmart it. If we don't outsmart it, we'll continue to ignore the long-term consequences whenever there is short-term pleasure available. Here's our problem in a nutshell: we are biologically programmed to eat whatever is around us, and we are usually surrounded by food. What a situation! To lose weight, we'll want to deal with this problem head on.

CHANGING OUR FOOD ENVIRONMENT

So what can we do to stop this strong, innate tendency to respond to food cues in our environment? One thing we can do is control our food environment at home. Although many of us eat out more frequently than ever, we still eat a large portion of our diet at home. Home is where we typically relax for the evening. For many of us, relaxing equates to eating. The degree to which we can change our home environment varies with each of us. Obviously, some of us have more control over our food environment than others. It may be possible for many of us to change our environment so that we are surrounded by fewer cues and therefore less temptation to eat. For all of us, however, and especially for those of us unable to change our home/food environment, it is extremely important to be aware of the food in our homes if we want to lose weight. Changing our home food environment will make a huge dent in our eating and help us lose weight. By simply not having tempting food around us, we increase our odds of eating a much healthier diet and attaining our goal of weight loss.

The primary problem with changing our home food environment is that most of us do not live alone. We think of the food in our cupboards as not being there for "us," but instead for "them". It is common to hear, "I don't want to deprive 'them' of the foods they love because of my issue." Although seemingly self-sacrificing, it is anything but that.

Eating food together has always been a way of bonding. Often, the only time all family members are in the same room is when they eat together. Food is also the focus of celebrations and festivities. Few rooms are as active as the kitchen. We even design homes with "open floor plans" that brings the warmth of the kitchen to the rest of the home. The food environment and the social environment can't be separated, although it might not seem that way when we sit alone clutching our bowl of no added sugar ice cream. Our food and our social environment that involves food can be difficult to manage when our goal is to lose weight. Yet even when trying to lose weight, we still want to appreciate the social importance food has in our lives, and continue to enjoy get-togethers where there is food. We don't want to give up these important events, and we don't have to. However, we do want strategies and tips that help us cope with having food around, and this includes dealing with the tasty images of food beckoning and enticing us in commercials. We'll take a closer look at this challenge latter and come up with some recommendations that have been successful and comfortable for many of us.

Food Helps Us Feel Better

It is difficult to talk about our food environment without slipping into a discussion of our social environment—food and socializing are intimately linked. Similarly, food and the workings of our mind (psychology) are also intimately linked. We are persuaded to eat for psychological reasons: Eating can change our attitude, feeling, and mood almost instantly, and in the most amazing ways. Although food's ability to affect our psychology is chemically based, our thoughts and behavior involved in eating are considered part of our psychology. If we have a drug that makes us feel good, we'd say the effect of the drug is biochemical, pure and simple. Although the desire might be chemically based, our decision concerning when, how often, and how much of the drug we take is psychological because it involves awareness and decision making. Our ideas and decisions determine our behavior. The concept that our thoughts determine our behavior is at the heart of the cognitive behavioral approach, the approach used in this book. The drug analogy isn't all that far off actually, and if we continue with the analogy, food is a multipurpose drug: it releases dopamine, which gives us "aah" moments," decreases our anxiety by helping us relax, perks us up, and feels satisfying and rewarding. Those are all wonderful! If food was illegal, we'd be on street corners trying to score a nickel bag of decadent chocolate! It is so darn good and so readily available, many of us use it to balance our emotional lives. If we had to stalk our food for hours, it would be much less a problem for us. If eating too much food didn't make us fat, we'd have no problem.

Too often, we eat because we are overly anxious or depressed, and we don't want our emotional stabilizers taken away from us. Why would we? We eat to deal with our feelings, and our feelings come from our thoughts; so if we can change our thoughts, we can change the urge to overeat. Recognizing and changing our thoughts is an essential part of a successful, permanent solution to weight loss. Further, certain patterns of thoughts are related to depression and anxiety, and as we begin to change those thoughts, anxiety and depression symptoms recede. Losing weight and feeling better emotionally go hand-in-hand. Of course, we'll want to stack the deck in our favor and find other ways to compensate for the satisfaction we got from overeating. We'll also want to build up our reward system to give us further incentive not to overeat. And hey, it is not like we're going without satisfying food! If you eat the right foods, you can still have satisfying meals and snacks as well as tame your appetite. Subsequent chapters will help you understand your unique psychology, how it influences your overeating, and what to do about it.

If you want to lose weight, keep it off, and be happy doing it, you'll want the advantage of using every resource available. You'll soon discover how to (1) control your biochemistry (specifically blood sugar levels), (2) control your food and social environment and, (3) deal with the psychological aspects of why you overeat. We are all different and will be influenced by the above three influences in different proportions. We're all playing with the same deck, but we've all been dealt a different hand. Fortunately, we don't have to embark on our weight loss mission alone. There are many professionals out there who want to help us. They are waiting to be asked, and are potential allies. Assembling an effective weight loss team is very important. It is time to introduce you to the professionals who are applying for membership to your team. Think of them as a smorgasbord of professionals (pardon the expression)!

☆　☆　☆

Chapter 4

HOW TO BUILD THE BEST SUPPORT TEAM

We are bombarded by a number of forces that contribute to our weight gain and sabotage our efforts to lose weight. These forces encourage us to overeat, and our scales taunt us with evidence of their success. Sure, we've had nibbles of success on crash diets, but victory was short-lived or required too great a sacrifice. We want more help. Fortunately, help is available.

When attacked, it is natural to be defensive. Common sense tells us to prepare to respond to each type of attack, and we have three to respond to: biochemistry, environmental cues to eat, and psychological pressure. If we limit ourselves to thwarting one or two of the forces, we might win a battle or two, but we won't win the war. Just as each conventional war is unique, so too is our own personal war against the forces making us overweight and diabetic. Although we are all attacked by the same forces, we all have a unique combination of those forces impacting us. Further, we all have our own distinctive way of dealing with challenges.

When we come to realize our old ways of losing weight and reversing our diabetes have proven unsuccessful, it is reassuring to know there are specialists available to help us. Think of them as specialized consultants or advisors. You pick and choose your consultants based upon your own personal wants and preferences. It's your body, your life, and your battle, so you are therefore the leader of your team. You don't have to know any of the answers to your questions as long as you surround yourself by people who do.

KNOW YOUR ENEMY

Far too many of us believe we are the enemy—or something deep down in us is the problem: We're too lazy, or we lack willpower, self-control, or sufficient self-respect! Baloney! Your mission to lose weight is not a fault-finding mission. Your enemy is not you. We are people with fat, not fat people. Losing weight is not about losing a part of your sense of your "self". You do not have to defend your weight or find excuses for it. However, you do want to discover the underlying reasons why you've accumulated excess weight. Once you understand your enemy—the forces that compel you to overeat—you can develop a sound strategy and outsmart them. Again, the enemy is not you, it is the fat that has already invaded your territory and has started to physically destroy you.

WATCH YOUR STEP!

Before we continue, it's time to clear the air on an important but rather personal matter: Word has it (gossip travels, you know) that you've been caught cavorting with the enemy on at least more than one occasion! Yes, rumor has it that you've used your weight to get out of some chores as well as justify some rather "bad" behavior. One unnamed and occasionally reliable source has even reported overhearing you mutter, "I might as well eat this, I'm fat already!" Remember, you are about to become a leader of a specialized team, so straighten up and watch your step! On a more reassuring note, if your weight has provided you some degree of protection from the stresses in life, and there is a good chance it has (even if you don't know exactly how yet), you will not lose the protection you need to cope with life. Actually, you will be trading up and discovering better ways to protect yourself. Successful long-term weight loss is about adding to your life, not taking things away from it. You will see yourself grow, not in girth, but in happiness and contentment. Success is yours if you choose foods that work with your biochemistry to reduce hunger while still providing satisfaction. Find non-food ways to provide you with the psychological comfort and excitement you desire; and take control of your food environment to reduce temptation. You can do it.

YOUR POTENTIAL TEAM SPECIALISTS

Your weight loss team members are those specialists you engage because of their expertise: doctors, psychologists, dietitians, etc. Some professionals, we all know, are better than others. Therefore, when possible, try to select and not settle. You can also discharge them at will. Remember you are in charge and in control, so don't be afraid of your power. You can successfully lead if you:

1. Are open to new ideas. This requires being humble and not defensive. It is easier said than done. You probably already know that.
2. Are wise enough to get the most out of the experts you assemble. In our case, this also sometimes means being an outstanding patient, client, or student. Yes, you can be a leader, a student, and a patient all at the same time. Remember: just as there are outstanding doctors, there are also outstanding patients. Be one.
3. Listen to the experts, even if you don't always like what they have to say. Everyone wants to help; it is just that some are more skilled at it than others. Be open to the advice of experts even if you don't always have the background or training to be able to fully evaluate their recommendations. Remember if you knew how to get out of this mess alone, you wouldn't be looking for help.
4. Be willing to replace experts who don't perform up to your standards. In other words, your team members are your consultants, but it is still your war.

If you know a professional who has expertise in diabetes *and* how to lose weight, and if the specialist is able and willing to evaluate, plan, coordinate, and oversee your weight loss strategy with you (which includes consultation and treatment by other specialists), consider yourself lucky…very lucky. Take the time to search for one and be willing to travel a fair distance. If you have access to a comprehensive treatment center, it is almost like one-stop shopping; it has many advantages, so consider taking advantage of it. One of the greatest benefits of a team approach is having better communication between team members, especially if they share the same treatment files. Even if you are fortunate enough to have access to a specialized team, you can still use the following information to help you get the most out of this type of specialty care…so keep reading.

Unfortunately, most of us do not have access to such a specialty service. Consequently, you will have to coordinate and manage some of the care yourself. Don't be intimidated by this. It is doable, very doable, if you know how to go about it. We are all different, and the help each of us requires is unique; therefore, you must assemble a team of specialists suited to your own particular situation. However, it might be premature at this point to decide what specialists you want, because like a savvy diner, you will want to read the whole menu before you make your selections. By the way, the specialists available to you on today's menu are all available a la carte:

CERTIFIED DIABETES EDUCATOR

A certified diabetes educator (CDE) can be a nurse, a registered dietitian, or any other healthcare professional certified as diabetes educators. Be sure they cover the basics of diabetes with you. A fundamental understanding of diabetes is a must for all of us. Information covered only a few years back can become outdated, leading many of us to use archaic terms and even misunderstand such basics as the definition of what is meant by low blood sugar. For example, even the term "complex carbohydrates" is no longer used by the American Diabetes Association! This book does not cover the basics, because there are plenty available that do an excellent job.

PSYCHOLOGISTS

There are many types of psychologists, but the ones we are most interested in are clinical psychologists. They work with patients in a therapeutic setting and treat a wide range of mental health issues and disorders. Anxiety and depression are the most common problems encountered by those of us with diabetes and obesity. Both depression and anxiety can get in the way of our efforts to lose weight. If we're depressed, we probably don't have the energy or enthusiasm to take on the challenge of losing weight. Feeling depressed, chronically sad, hopeless, or helpless, zaps the energy we want to get the job done—be it weight loss or anything else. Losing weight is not an easy job; it takes consistent effort. If you are depressed, even mildly, you may not give yourself a fair shot at losing weight. Psychologists can evaluate you for depression and treat it so you're better prepared to take on challenges such as weight loss. Now, don't worry about diagnosing yourself if you are not sure if you are depressed or not. There are a host of reasons both medical and psychological for someone to feel lethargic or depressed. For example, diabetes itself often mimics the symptoms of depression and disorientation. Teasing out depressive symptoms from the symptoms caused by diabetes is a difficult task. A clinical psychologist can evaluate you for depression and/or any other mental health issue that might impede your weight loss efforts. Like depression, excessive anxiety can also sabotage your efforts to lose weight. If you feel anxious or "stressed out," you are less likely to succeed at consistent weight loss.

Depression and anxiety are sometimes directly related to our eating. We might be eating to help us control uncomfortable feelings such as sadness or anxiety. Now that you understand some of the amazing chemistry involved in hunger and eating, you can perhaps see how and why we commonly use food to keep some sort of emotional balance in our lives. If you have the opportunity to stand back and look at the patterns of your behavior with a professional, especially in regard to eating, you'll be well rewarded.

A psychologist's expertise goes beyond the treatment of depression and anxiety. They can also evaluate and treat other psychological problems such as bi-polar disorder (it used to be called manic-depression), substance abuse, family and relationship problems, etc.

When being overweight is combined with having diabetes and mental health issues, the most effective form of therapy is cognitive behavioral therapy. "Cognitive" refers to our thinking processes, and "behavioral" refers to the actions we take based on our thoughts. Cognitive behavioral therapy assists individuals in improving their moods or emotions, such as helping them cope more effectively with negative emotions. It uncovers distorted thinking patterns that produce negative mood states, such as anxiety and depression, and teaches individuals how to correct them. Cognitive behavioral therapy (CBT) helps motivate individuals to engage in healthy behaviors along with dissuading them from engaging in unhealthy ones. Research has consistently demonstrated that therapy, either individual or group therapy, in combination with any form of weight loss or diabetes management program, greatly improves outcomes for all participants. Give yourself the best odds at success. Why settle for anything less?

PSYCHIATRISTS

Sometimes cognitive behavioral therapy is not enough, and you might benefit from a medication such as an antidepressant or anti-anxiety medication. Psychologists cannot prescribe medication. Doctors such as internists frequently prescribe antidepressants and anti-anxiety medications, but it sometimes depends on the complexity of the presenting problem, the willingness and knowledge base of the physician, and their knowledge of the patient. Common practice aside, only a psychiatrist is specially trained to perform a comprehensive mental health evaluation and prescribe the appropriate psychotropic medication (a medication that treats mental disorders). Psychiatrists are aware of the latest treatment options, and can prescribe just the right medication or combination of medications to treat your specific diagnosis as well as specific symptoms. For example, even though two individuals might share the same diagnosis, such as depression, one might be highly anxious and unable to sleep, and the other might sleep all day. Such individuals may therefore benefit from different medications. Treatment is much more complex than some television ads suggest. Some psychiatrists also offer talk therapy, and a few even offer cognitive behavioral therapy.

INTERNISTS

Internists deal with the prevention, diagnosis, and treatment of adult diseases. They can provide non-surgical care for your weight loss, diabetes, and other health conditions. Before starting any weight loss program, you'll want to check with your primary care physician, often an internist. Your internist can complete a physical examination, review your medical history (including medication and surgical history), and determine if there are any health concerns related to your planned weight loss. They can also explore your desire, if any, for a weight loss medication, and check to be sure there are no contraindications before one is prescribed. Some internists also measure their patient's body composition via a BIA (bioelectrical impedance analysis) scale which measures body fat levels. For us, these scales are more accurate than conventional scales, because they provide more relevant information.

REGISTERED DIETITIANS (RD)

A registered dietitian (RD) can be an essential part of your team, because they can help you with your dietary strategy to lose weight and lower blood sugar levels. This is done through education about nutrition, meal planning, etc. Don't be surprised if the first step they take is to help you prevent binge eating. They can also help you plan your food intake, monitor your calories, as well as provide overall support. Your RD will also discuss physical activity and how it relates to your weight loss efforts. An RD is the only health care provider with professional training to do this.

EXERCISE PHYSIOLOGISTS

An exercise physiologist can evaluate your exercise requirements and your ability to safely engage in various exercises. They can evaluate cardiac risk, pain levels, and other factors that might influence the type and quality of exercise that becomes part of your routine. Physical activity treatment usually consists of group aerobic classes and use of aerobic equipment. The American Diabetes Association recommends aerobic exercise as the primary mode of exercise. If, due to medical conditions other than diabetes, aerobic exercise is not recommended, an exercise physiologist can help you develop an exercise program suited to your particular requirements.

CARDIOLOGISTS

Cardiologists are medical doctors who specialize in the heart and circulatory system. Cardiac (heart) failure is the leading cause of death for those of us with diabetes. This is due directly to the damage to our body, including our heart, caused by diabetes. A cardiologist assesses the present condition of your heart and circulatory system. This is accomplished by performing a physical examination, evaluating blood work, conducting a stress test, and reviewing X-rays and CT scans. The results can then be used by your cardiologist to provide treatment, if warranted. They can also share their findings with other members of your weight loss treatment team so your treatment never puts your heart or circulatory system at risk. Regardless of specialty and findings, always think of yourself as the middle man when it comes to sharing important information amongst the specialists on your team. Take nothing for granted. When it comes to any form of medical care, never assume one hand knows what the other hand is doing; never assume important information is passed from one specialist to another. Remember, you are the leader and the buck stops with you.

OPTHTHALMOLOGISTS

Ophthalmologists are medical doctors who diagnose and treat conditions of the eyes. Because those of us with diabetes often experience problems with our eyes, such as retinopathy (disorders of the retina), cataracts (opacity of the lens), and glaucoma (high fluid pressure in the eye), it is suggested that all of us with diabetes have our eyes examined regularly. Visual problems can lead to decreased physical activity as well as limit one's ability to gather information through reading, the Internet, television, etc. Unfortunately, ophthalmological degeneration often comes on slowly, so slowly in fact, that we are not fully aware our visual problems cause us to change our behavior to accommodate our failing eyesight. Just like people who blame friends and family for not talking loud enough when they start losing their hearing, visual impairments might fool us too. For example, we might start to avoid stairs because of the fear of tripping due to our lessened ability to see, or perhaps we will start to avoid locations other than very well-lighted areas (and blame the lighting). Similarly, we may find ourselves reading less, or straining harder when we do read and not stop to consider why.

ENDOCRINOLOGISTS

An endocrinologist is a medical doctor who evaluates and treats diabetes as well as other hormonal problems. Endocrinologists prescribe diabetes medication, and can tailor the medication to the unique requirements of each individual patient. Because some diabetes medications have the side effect of weight gain, an endocrinologist can balance the desire to lower blood sugar levels with the importance of losing weight. Although this can be quite complicated, endocrinologists are trained and experienced in prescribing just the right medications or combination of medications.

BARIATRIC SURGEONS

Bariatric physicians deal with the causes, prevention and treatment of obesity. As such, they are prepared to explain all the current surgical procedures available for weight loss. They are familiar with the effectiveness of the various procedures as well as the risks involved in weight loss surgery.

PULMONOLOGISTS

It is estimated that about 80% of us, specifically those of us who fall into the "obese" medical category, have untreated sleep apnea. Sleep apnea is a condition that causes abnormal pauses in breathing during sleep. There are a couple different types of sleep apnea, but the one we're interested in has to do with an obstruction to our airflow due to our extra weight. The pauses in breathing can last from seconds to minutes, and they can occur a few times an hour up to over thirty times an hour. Sleep apnea is a dangerous condition. It is especially harmful to our heart, and can interfere with weight loss, because the person with sleep apnea is often too fatigued and sleepy during the day to pay attention to weight loss activities. Fortunately, it can be treated by pulmonologists. It is diagnosed by conducting a sleep study. Talk to your physician to see if there is a benefit in consulting with a pulmonologist. Below are some, but not all, of the major symptoms of obstructive sleep apnea:

- Excessive daytime sleepiness or tiredness
- Not feeling refreshed in the morning
- Gasping or choking at night
- Snoring
- Problems with concentration and memory
- Personality or attitude changes
- Morning or nighttime headaches
- Sour taste or heartburn at night
- Swelling of the legs
- Sweating and/or chest pain at night
- Frequent nighttime urination
- Frequently waking up at night, or frequently tossing or turning

RADIOLOGISTS

Radiologists can provide the most accurate assessment of your body's composition and measure your progress. Typical weight scales do not do a good job of measuring progress on a daily basis. Keep in mind that we want to lose body fat, not just weight. Weight not only includes body fat, but also includes muscles and water.

PHYSIATRISTS

Physiatrists are medical doctors who specialize in physical medicine and rehabilitation; therefore, they are commonly called PMRs. They are also referred to as sports medicine physicians. They can evaluate you and identify any special requirements related to any underlying skeletal or muscular condition that may affect your ability to exercise.

PHYSICAL THERAPISTS

Physical therapists (PTs) treat health-related conditions in individuals with illnesses, injuries or conditions that limit their physical ability. They can provide treatment and develop exercises for individuals who are physically injured or impaired.

WHICH FORM OF ASSISTANCE IS RIGHT FOR YOUR WEIGHT LOSS?

There are many options on the above menu of specialists from which to choose, and it is hard to imagine anyone requiring all of them. You are going to have to make some choices, but some decisions can be made later. All choices are open to reconsideration. If you already have some ideas about whom you want on your team, good for you. Here are some things to keep in mind regarding your team selections:

- You want a starting point, so choose a professional from the list that gives you the best advantage of getting off to a good start. Choosing one with the greatest overview might help you decide on whom to include on your team. Alternatively, you can start with the professional you have grown to most trust. You can ask any of your specialists for suggestions on whom else to include in your team. It is fun to play dumb and ask anyway. You can then compare answers later. You might find some differences of opinion, but there's nothing wrong with that. It doesn't always mean one is right and one is wrong. Don't confuse opinions with facts (even though they are sometimes presented as such).

- If you have a clear idea where your major problem lies, put the appropriate specialist towards the top of your list. Just be open to being wrong about what you consider to be your major problem. You might think differently once you learn more and get professional opinions. For example, if you believe you are suffering from depression, see a psychologist if you believe you can address your problem by changing your behavior and gaining insight into your problem. If you believe you could benefit from an antidepressant, see a psychiatrist. If you know your diet is lousy, and you want to address that, be sure to place "registered dietitian" near the top of your list.

- You can change the list of specialists on your consulting team anytime you darn well please (unless you are dealing with health insurance gatekeepers or other limitations). You can even opt to consult with some of them just once if you want. In fact, as you learn more about your options, as well as your own status, you will probably want to add or remove some of the specialists. They are your consultants, and you can do what you want with them!

- Once you see a professional and have your preliminary list of specialists you would like on your team, see if there is a particular order in which you would like to initially consult with them. Unfortunately, due to insurance and scheduling limitations, you might not get them in the order you want. You'll deal with that the best you can. "Sweet talking" the person scheduling appointments never hurts, especially if you first go out of your way to learn their first name and appeal to their special powers to "make space" for special people. Threats to let the air out of their tires don't work. Schedulers always have the last laugh.

- Trust your gut. If you don't like someone whose specialty you want on your team, find a replacement for them. Just keep in mind that we often judge medical professionals almost exclusively on their bedside manner. Evaluating their clinical skills is next to impossible for most of us. Leave the evaluation of their expertise up to other professionals you trust. Don't forget to ask nurses for their opinions. They often have the best information and inside information. Opinions are best pried out of them by promising to keep your discussion confidential. They'll be flattered you asked them. Asking them who they would go to if they had your problem is a safe way to start.

- Put the time, research and energy into your weight loss that you would for someone you love or admire. This may sound like common sense, but it is far from common practice. Strange, isn't it?

- Be sure to understand your medical insurance limitations, preapprovals, etc. If you have an insurance plan with a "gatekeeper," be sure to make them your new best friend. Because "obesity" costs insurance companies dearly, they may be much more supportive of your weight loss efforts than you expect. Even Medicare approves behavioral treatment for obesity.

- Some medical insurance companies (or plans) provide discounts to exercise centers, so don't overlook this. They like healthy subscribers, because they don't cost as much to keep alive.

OH NO, NOT ANOTHER ANALOGY!

You've been encouraged to think of yourself as the leader of a team of specialists, and consider them advisors and consultants. Help comes in many forms, and some of the specialists have things that might help you. You are probably already somewhat familiar with most of them, but they are worth reviewing. Please remove your leader hat and change into your swimwear...yes, you read correctly... swimwear!

Losing weight and keeping it off is like swimming across an ocean. Let's make it the Atlantic Ocean. As you depart from the sandy shores of upscale Miami Beach, you will have the option to take along some swim gear. Some swim gear might aid your swim across the ocean, but there may also be some downsides to each of your gear options. Consistency of approach, however, is the key to permanent weight loss. So keep this in mind when reviewing your options.

Swimming a long distance, like weight loss, entails a steady, daily effort. If you go too fast, you'll burn out. If you take too long a break when swimming, the natural flow of the current will wash you back ashore. You'll not look your best when you wash back up on the beautiful beach with sand in your hair and seaweed between your teeth. When you start and stop swimming, you lose your "glide," your forward momentum. The same holds true for weight loss and diabetes management. Getting started is the hardest step, and if you start and stop, you are making the process harder. Certainly you can recall all those terrible Monday mornings when you were on a "diet" and "cheated" over the weekend. In addition to having to start all over again Monday morning (ugh), chances are you also felt guilty when you were "cheating" during the weekend anyway! Stopping and starting is an unsound strategy, both biologically and psychologically; it keeps you in a constant on and off dieting mode rather than allowing you to make a permanent lifestyle change. Below are some aids, comparable to swim gear, that are available to you for weight loss:

WEIGHT LOSS MEDICATIONS

Swimming across the Atlantic using a weight loss medication is like using arm flotation devices, sometimes known by the brand name "Swimmies". When you get tired, the arm devices help you stay afloat. On the downside, they can become irritating, not unlike the side-effects of weight loss medications. Sooner or later, most people discard their arm floats. If you use the arm floats at the expense of learning how to swim, you too will inevitably drift back to the shore. If, however, you are sharp enough to use the medication as a jump-start, and not a long-term solution, you will be well on your way to making a lasting change. This is not to say that a medication won't one day be developed for long-term use. Just don't hold your breath…especially when swimming!

LAP-BAND SURGERY

Having lap-band surgery is like paddling across the ocean using a surfboard. The increased floatation of the board allows you to get more glide with each stroke. You can take breaks and keep on moving; but without constant vigilance, you too will drift back. It takes a lot of work to paddle across the Atlantic, and a lap-band can make the swim easier.

GASTRIC BYPASS

Having a gastric bypass is like crossing the ocean in a rowboat. Whereas the big waves push the arm floaters and surfboarders back toward shore, the rowboat is substantial enough to more easily slice through the waves. A gastric bypass can help you move forward amidst an overly abundant food environment; but, like the oars of a boat that give out halfway across, so does a bypass. Unfortunately, most people who have this procedure don't lose 100% of their excess weight. They stay adrift but only about half-way to their goal. However, if the procedure saves their life, it is well worth it.

OTHER WEIGHT LOSS PROGRAMS

Certainly, if you have the willpower, losing weight entirely "on your own" is possible. It is done every day. People will even respect and applaud your success. Popular television shows often demonstrate this type of dramatic weight loss. Most people attempting to lose weight this way, however, are attracted to inexpensive, short-sighted programs that don't keep the weight off in the long run. They usually don't account for the complication of also having to deal with diabetes or the desire to make a lifestyle change. Approaching weight loss and diabetes control from all fronts—biological, psychological and environmental/social—gives us the best chance of long-term success.

PERMANENT WEIGHT LOSS REQUIRES A LIFESTYLE CHANGE

To make it across the ocean when your surfboard, rowboat, or arm floats stop working, you will want to continue swimming to the far shore. Similarly, you will want to change the way you eat each day to make it to the far shore. You'll be swimming for a long time, because you are not going to reach your goal overnight. You want a pace you can sustain in the long run, and to lose weight requires a lifestyle change. It means that you'll have to change the way you think, feel, and behave about food and eating in order to reach your goal and relish your accomplishment. If you can pick up bad habits, you can certainly choose to pick up a few good ones. You will no longer have to give that blank stare when someone advises you to, "Don't diet; change your lifestyle." This is annoying advice if you don't have the tools and support to accomplish this change.

If you get the right help, you can be successful. It is done every day. It is not easy, but it is certainly within your ability. The rewards (beyond better health) are extremely gratifying. Your physique will change, your self-regard will change, and the way people treat you will change. What an enormous personal accomplishment it will be! No one—absolutely no one—who has accomplished this feat says it wasn't worth the effort. Remember this when the going gets rough. Now, slip out of your swimwear until the next analogy.

No doubt you are itching to learn what to eat to tame your extreme appetite. Eating the right combinations of carbohydrates will help you do this. You can decrease your appetite, better control your blood sugar levels, and still feel full and satisfied after your meals and snacks. Amazing!

Chapter 5

THE HUNGER-BUSTING APPROACH TO EATING

You already have a good idea why it is so darn hard to lose weight when you have type 2 diabetes by simply remembering some of the crazy biochemistry involved in hunger, blood sugar levels, and fat storage. To bust your hunger to a level where you can lose weight, you'll have to outsmart your biochemistry. To do that, you'll first want a more thorough understanding of the biochemical forces previously mentioned. To start with, you'll want to understand the different types of foods you eat and how you react to them. You'll also want to become better acquainted with your old friend, insulin.

INSULIN

Those of us with diabetes, and even pre-diabetes, initially produce too much ineffective insulin. As diabetes progresses, insulin production diminishes and we have high blood sugar levels. Insulin is a hormone produced by the beta cells of the pancreas gland. The pancreas is located near our stomach. Insulin's main function is to take food out of the blood stream and store it in cells throughout our body. The nutrition it removes from the blood stream can be in the form of sugar (glucose), fat or protein. The cells where this nutrition is stored can be muscle cells, fat cells, or other types of body tissue.

When sugar enters our blood stream rapidly, as is the case when we eat white bread or candy, our pancreas senses this sudden rise in sugar. Unless our body's blood sugar level is abnormally low, it does not like a rapid increase in blood sugar. When it does sense a rapid rise, it releases insulin to decrease the high level of sugar in our blood. The insulin grabs the sugar and stores it in cells—in our case, usually in fat cells.

THE DIABETIC'S DILEMMA

A diabetic's blood sugar level can begin to creep up higher for a variety of reasons: genetics, lack of exercise, and overconsumption. In all people, diabetic or not, the beta cells produce and release insulin in response to high blood sugar levels. Usually, insulin binds to our body's cells—think of this as the insulin hooking onto, or docking with them. Once bound to our cells, the insulin grabs the sugar out of the blood stream and stores it inside the cells. This "grab and store" process gets screwed up in diabetes and pre-diabetes.

In diabetes and pre-diabetes, the insulin that is bound to our cells doesn't work properly, because our fat cells become obnoxious and send out mean-spirited messages (in the form of toxins) to other cells warning them not to bind with the insulin. With our body's cells refusing to bind with the insulin due to badmouthing, insulin builds up in our bodies. Unfortunately, this insulin rejection is happening behind the back of our pancreas (not the smartest organ in our body). Sensing something is amiss, however, but not fully understanding what's wrong, our pancreas decides to come on stronger and pump even more insulin into our bloodstream! In diabetics and even pre-diabetics, this results in abnormally high blood sugar levels. Fortunately, the dim-witted pancreas eventually allows things to get back to normal, and our blood sugar level goes back down.

Bad for us is that due to all the extra insulin in our system, our body goes into a "storage mode". This makes sense if you think of your great, great ancestors who had to gorge and fill up on food during periods when it was plentiful. When they gorged, the intent was to store the nutrition for later use, and not burn it up while still gorging. To burn up the extra nutrition while gorging would have been stupid… or in polite circles, "maladaptive". It is not unlike a bear storing up fat for the long winter. But back to humans, and specifically those of us with diabetes, once this "storage mode" switch is hit, most (if not almost all) of what we eat gets packed into fat cells. Now, here comes the real kicker: because our body is in a storage mode and grabs most of the sugar from our blood stream, there is a good chance our blood sugar level will dip. Remember that your brain runs primarily on sugar, and if your body is storing it away, it is out of reach of the brain. What's a poor brain to do? It does the obvious: it sends out signals which we experience as cravings for more sugar! After additional sugar is consumed, insulin will grab the newly ingested sugar. Once again, our brain will be left in a deprived state! The brain, in turn, sends out yet more craving signals all over again! And you've been trying to fight this chemical warfare with willpower alone? Really?

In some of us with severe cases of type 2 diabetes (meaning we are highly insulin resistant), the blood sugar level and insulin levels can *both* remain elevated for long periods. In this case, the pancreas is refusing to give up, and the beta cells just keep pumping out insulin in overdrive. Like most things in overdrive too long, damage can occur. In our case, our beta cells can die, and our diabetes can become much, much worse. With intent to alert rather than scare, we all want to be aware of the consequences of not taking proper care of our diabetes. When people are "scared" their decision making ability is often not at its best. They'll end up going on a crash diet, trying to live on shakes, or dabble with their medication without their doctor's approval.

The process explained above is so important it is worth repeating, so here it goes:

1. People with diabetics have higher blood sugar levels.
2. Insulin is secreted by the beta cells of our pancreas gland to reduce the sugar level.
3. Insulin docks (or attaches) to our body's cells.
4. Our fat cells send out warning to other cells to reject the insulin.
5. Our pancreas doesn't notice this and keeps sending out more insulin.
6. Our blood sugar level continues to rise.
7. A "storage mode" is triggered.
8. Blood sugar levels eventually drop.
9. When our blood sugar levels drop, our brains demand more sugar.
10. We listen to our brains and eat sugars (short-acting carbs).
11. We become frustrated and curse each time we step on the scale.

Realizing what goes on in our body, you can now see why it is so easy for us to pack on the pounds and have such a hard time losing weight. It is as if we're fighting with our own bodies, and in some ways we are. And because we can't "will" this powerful biochemistry away, or ignore our own brain signals for any reasonable length of time, we come to the conclusion we lack willpower. Remember that old "excuse" for being heavy, you know: "I have a glandular problem"? Apparently, many of us who used that explanation were not inaccurate after all! But before we feel completely vindicated and start waving our books in the air, we're reminded there are still some other "contributing factors" to our weight problem…as if biochemistry isn't enough!

Fortunately, there are a couple of ways of break out of the crazy insulin production and fat storage mode. The first is an eating plan with controlled amounts of simple carbohydrates, and the second one is exercise.

CARBOHYDRATES

Carbohydrates (or carbs for short) are chemical compounds formed mostly by plants. They provide fuel to our bodies. Carbohydrates include sugars, starches and cellulose. The most important form of carbohydrate is glucose, a simple sugar. Glucose is the energy source of nearly all known living things. When you test your blood sugar level, you are testing your blood glucose level (BG). Foods contain various amounts of carbohydrates; some foods have more carbohydrates than others, and some release their fuel faster than others.

For illustration, carbohydrates are *usually* placed into one of two categories: short-acting (simple) and long-lasting (complex) carbs. Short-acting or simple carbohydrates elevate our blood sugar level quickly, and long-lasting carbohydrates take longer to break down into glucose after we eat them. Long-acting carbs are sometimes referred to as "complex" carbs, but the term "complex carbs" is so misused in advertising, we'll avoid using it. Actually, foods containing carbohydrates fall along a wide range (or continuum) from simple on one extreme, to very long-lasting on the other. Foods can fall anywhere between these two extremes.

A diet low in short-acting carbohydrates does not elevate our blood sugar quickly, and because of this, the pancreas doesn't dispense insulin beyond that which is needed for our basic functioning. Depending on the severity of our diabetes, once we start a low carbohydrate diet, it can take days to decrease our blood sugar and insulin levels, so don't expect it to happen overnight. People often give up before really getting into it, because the pancreas continues to pump out high levels of insulin in preparation for high blood sugar levels (remember it is a slow learner). Unfortunately, with all that insulin in our system and minimal blood sugar, our blood sugar level often drops too low. This is called "hypoglycemia" (notice the *hypo*). When we become hypoglycemic, we often try to correct the problem by overeating simple carbohydrates. This can raise our blood sugar level too high, to a "hyperglycemic" level (notice it becomes *hyper*). When this happens, we are on the diabetes rollercoaster again. We want to put the brakes on this hazardous ride.

EXERCISE

Exercise is as close as we get to a "switch" that turns off pancreatic insulin production. Within ten minutes of moderate exercise such as a brisk walk, the pancreas drastically decreases the amount of insulin being produced, and our body begins to use the sugar in the blood stream for energy. At about the twenty-minute mark, your body burns through the sugar in your blood and then starts using body fat as its primary source of energy. Yes, the energy stored in fat cells actually starts getting burned up! Voila, you go from a "storage mode" to a "burning mode," and all within about twenty minutes! This is so encouraging that it is understandable if you decide to put this book down and take a brisk walk right now!

With exercise and a diet limited in simple carbohydrates, the pancreas is effectively "reset" and insulin production grinds to a slow crawl. At this slower insulin production pace:

- Your body can utilize fat for energy;
- Your blood sugar/insulin pathway is repaired;
- Your blood sugar levels decrease; and
- The disease process of diabetes slows down and in some cases stops entirely.

Now, admit this is nothing less than amazing!

Before you embark on "resetting" your pancreas through diet and exercise, remember the old warning about, "too much of a good thing". We diabetics cannot eat a diet without at least some simple carbs. This is because our pancreas is producing too much insulin (which is called hyperinsulinemia). If we don't consume simple carbs, our blood sugar levels can drop too low at first. This is why it is so extremely uncomfortable to continue eating a diet free of simple carbs, regardless of their fashionable names. If we jump into a very low or no-carb diet, we pull the sugar out of our blood and muscles, but there's only about 2,000 calories stored there. When that runs out, and if we are still producing insulin (which is highly likely), our blood sugar level will plummet. We know how our brain feels about falling blood sugar levels! We'll be hypoglycemic and our brain will be screaming for a lot of delicious, decadent food to get our sugar level back up. This is why the "no simple carbs" diets usually last only two days.

CONTROL YOUR BLOOD SUGAR AND LOSE WEIGHT TOO

You can lower your blood sugar to a safer level and lose weight with the same diet. Many of us fear having to adhere to a special diet that is both complicated and depriving. A good diet for diabetics is neither. It is a diet with which you can live, and one that is acceptable and satisfying enough to become part not only of your lifestyle but your family's as well.

It is now necessary that you add another type of carb to your list and begin to think of carbs as being, "short, medium, or long". This classification is your new framework for future meal planning and food intake. You'll want to understand the difference between these carb types, and combine them correctly to bring about hunger management, weight loss and control of your blood sugar levels.

Carbs are in everything from broccoli, to ice-cream. Carbs are in all plant matter, from the seedling of a stalk of wheat to the white bread that results after processing and cooking the mature wheat grains. Carbs are in everything from candy, on one extreme, to kale on the other. One type of carb will raise your blood sugar and promote weight gain, and another type will have minimal, virtually unnoticeable effects on your blood sugar and will not result in weight gain. Making this dietary alteration will change your life—so much so that you can measure the results in pounds and inches.

MEET YOUR CARBS

Please meet your carbs: short, medium and long. Think of them this way:

1. Short-acting: Think *short-lasting or short-term*. When eaten, it takes them a *short* time to get your blood sugar levels to rise. They hit fast, hit hard and spike your blood sugar. They are highly pleasurable, and provide the *short-term* satisfaction you crave. They provoke insulin production. Also think of *"short-term"* carbs as *"simple"* carbs. These two terms are interchangeable.
2. Medium-acting: Think *medium-lasting* or *medium-term*. These carbs are somewhere between short and long-acting carbs; they are *midrange* carbs. They don't have the immediate spike found in short carbs. Instead, they provide a more *moderate* rise in blood sugar, and this *modest* rise extends for a longer period of time. When you think *medium* carbs, think *milk* products.
3. Long-acting: Think *long-lasting* or *long-term*. These wonderful carbs release their energy slowly over a *long* period of time. They are the "time-released" form of carbs. When you think of *"long"* carbs, think vegetables. Here's a recap before a more complete discussion of each:

Short-Acting Carbohydrates or Simple Carbohydrates
They provide sugar immediately.
They take a few seconds to an hour to raise your blood sugar level.
They provide taste, satisfaction and happiness!

Medium Acting Carbohydrates
They're in low-fat milk products.
They raise blood sugar levels 1 to 2 hours after eating
and they last longer.
They sit heavily in the stomach and provide feelings
of fullness while tasting slightly sweet.

Long Acting Carbohydrates
They're in non-starchy vegetables.
They raise your blood sugar in 3 to 5 hours, and
last longest without spikes.
They expand the stomach and provide immediately feelings of
fullness.

SHORT-ACTING CARBS OR SIMPLE CARBS

Simple carbs are in all fruit, bread, and starchy vegetables such as peas, beans, corn, and potatoes. We have been led a bit astray by the marketing and promotion of "whole grains". They've been presented as something more akin to broccoli rather than a slice of white bread. Nothing could be further from the truth. Grain products are composed of simple carbs. Further, the majority of products being touted as "whole grain" products do not consist entirely of "whole grains". Check the list of ingredients on the product. Often, you'll find they have refined flour as the primary ingredient, and have some seeds and sprouts thrown in so it can live up to its name or have eye appeal. It doesn't matter if the flour is enriched, non-enriched, stone-milled, bleached, unbleached, or plays the banjo and sings folk tunes—it makes absolutely no difference. Even if a product is *really* made completely of whole grains, it still will raise your blood sugar within the hour. Whole grains fare only slightly better than products made from refined flour. Whole grains are "the best of the worst" when it comes to simple carbs, but think of refined flour products as "the worst of the worst". Now, be sure to be seated for this one: flour raises our blood sugar faster than candy and sweets! Who would have thought!

Fruit also contains simple sugars. Fruit is considered by most to be a healthy food with no harmful effects. Although it usually has more vitamins and less fat and sugar than "junk food," hence its reputation as a healthy food. Fruit can be an unhealthy choice for diabetics. In fact, fruits like bananas can often raise your blood sugar levels extremely fast. Not all fruit is equal, however: fruits like apples typically raise the blood sugar level at a slower pace than bananas, but nevertheless, apples still manage to accomplish this within the hour. A general rule of thumb is that fruits found near the equator raise blood sugar levels faster than those naturally growing farther from the equator. For example, bananas, oranges, and pineapples are naturally found in warm weather climates, and they raise blood sugar levels more rapidly than apples, strawberries, and raspberries that are found in cooler climates. Also, when we eat the skin with the fruit, like with an apple, our blood sugar is less likely to rise as quickly.

Simple carbohydrates enter our blood stream the quickest. In response, our pancreas releases the most insulin in order to get the sugar (glucose) out of our blood stream. If left in the blood stream, glucose can cause damage to blood vessels, nerves and organs. This removal system would work fine if our insulin didn't store the sugar as fat. Those jokes about certain desserts going directly to our thighs are not so absurd or funny anymore, are they? Many a true thing is said in jest.

Actually, the joke is *really* on us; it doesn't end with the chocolate cake attaching itself to Mrs. Jones's thighs. Instead, it starts a viscous cycle that goes as follows:

The Insulin Spike Cycle

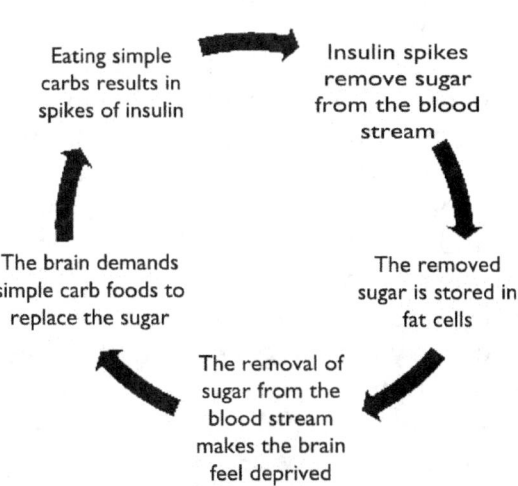

Fortunately, there are great alternatives to the simple carbs: medium-acting carbs and slow-acting (long-lasting) carbs. The longer lasting the carb, the less the amount of insulin is produced. Consequently, less sugar is stored as fat. Nice, very nice!

MEDIUM-ACTING CARBS

Medium carbs are milk products and "milk-like" products. Their sugars enter our system at a slower pace than simple carbs. Because of this, the pancreas pumps out less insulin and you get less storage as fat. Milk carbs are very hard for your body to break down, so much so that some people have an especially difficult time with this, and are considered "lactose intolerant". However, don't make the mistake of eating high-fat dairy products like butter or cheese and assume that this is giving you a medium sugar. It doesn't quite work that way. Unfortunately, as the fat content goes up, the milk sugar level goes down. You don't want that extra fat anyway, so now you have two reasons to avoid them. Products like skim milk, no-fat or low-fat cheese, and sugar free puddings made of skim milk all fall into the category of good, medium carbs. Milk-like products also include foods like soy and tofu. Lentils also fall into this category…don't ask why.

LONG-TERM CARBS

Vegetables do not taste good, or in the very least, they do not taste as good as scrumptious, simple carbohydrates. This does not apply, of course, to that tempting mélange of vegetables secreted under an abundant serving of rich, glorious hollandaise sauce, or even a fresh veggie drowning in butter. When was the last time you sat down to a head of broccoli and said "ooh" and "aah" or celebrated with a birthday cabbage? (If you did, you might want to keep quiet about it.) On the other hand, how did you react to that last slice of homemade pie you had? Your "oohs" and "aahs" were probably heard by your neighbors! You made sounds that can't be spelled, didn't you? You were delighted, because simple sugars gave you hedonistic pleasure (sensual pleasures); they are extremely satisfying. Vegetables, at best, get accolades like "fresh," "nice and crispy" or "juicy". They simply do not make us gasp in delight or speak in tongues. If they did, we wouldn't have an eating problem. Re-conceptualize vegetables as medicine if you want—something you ingest for your health. Rid yourself of the notion that whatever you eat is supposed to taste great. Not everything good for you is tasty. This simple thought never occurs to many of us.

Non starchy vegetables sit in your stomach and place pressure on your stomach walls producing a feeling of fullness. Vegetables are broken down slowly and give you energy three to five hours from the time you eat them. You'll have a healthier blood sugar level many hours after eating vegetables. Don't think of vegetables' purpose as existing to provide you with hedonistic pleasure; think of vegetables as you do exercise. Exercise isn't necessarily pleasurable either, unless, perhaps, it involves a sport or distraction—then it's pleasurable for a different reason. Despite what your exercise obsessed friends might say, especially about endorphins, nobody has pure pleasure while exercising. They do not say "ooh" and "aah" on the treadmill (unless it is groans of discomfort). Exercise and eating vegetables provide a form of pleasure called mastery pleasure. Mastery pleasure occurs when there is little about the activity that brings physiological or hedonistic pleasure, but instead, brings pleasure from mastering the activity, from achieving something. Success feels great, but it is a psychological pleasure or satisfaction, not a sensual or hedonistic one. You will experience mastery pleasure if you change your diet and step off the self-defeating simple carb rollercoaster. What an accomplishment it will be! It could indeed be "sweet success".

RESTRUCTURE YOUR DIET

When you restructure your meals and snacks into the SML (short-medium-long) carb framework (we'll call it SML from now on), losing weight and making your blood sugars smaller will be a cinch. All you want to do is eat an unlimited amount of very long carbs, a fair amount of no or low-fat milk products, and limit your simple carbs from between 100 and 200 calories per meal or snack (that's between 25 grams and 50 grams).

YOU DON'T HAVE TO GIVE UP TASTY FOODS

Although you will be eating vegetables that are not on the top of your list of tasty treats, you do not have to give up tasty food. As a matter of fact, you are encouraged…yes, encouraged to eat some simple carbs! Simple carbs provide the taste you crave and the sugar your brain demands. Remember your brain runs optimally on sugar, not protein or fat. We want happy brains, and eating carbs makes our brains happy. Because our brains seek happiness, our food taste preferences usually involve simple carbs in one form or another, such as bread, candy, cookies, pastries, etc. The hedonistic pleasure we experience when eating simple carbs is therefore downright good for us. Pleasure is a good thing, it makes our overall satisfaction and happiness levels go up and our sadness go down. Although the gratifying effects of simple carbs may be fleeting, they are something we all want and certainly deserve. Therefore, simple carbs *are not* to be left out of your diet! Eating too many simple carbs, however, is "too much of a good thing".

YOU DON'T HAVE TO GIVE UP FEELING FULL

Although "too much of a good thing" holds true for simple carbs, it doesn't for medium or long-acting carbs. Milk sugars (medium carbs) sit in our stomachs and provide us with feelings of fullness. If you don't believe everything you read, imagine trying to drink a gallon of skim milk in one sitting. You'll probably want to warn those around you there is a chance you will become physically sick. There's money to be made betting against you. On the other hand, no one would bet against you if you tried to make a few extra bucks by getting people to wager that you couldn't drink a gallon of soda. You could undoubtedly do that, and after, ask for a thirst quencher just to rub it in! That's because simple sugars fly through our stomach, whereas milk sugars do not. Milk sugars help us feel full, satiated, and satisfied.

PROTEIN IS OKAY, BUT BE MINDFUL OF FATS

Researchers used to think that when blood sugar levels went low, diabetics would crave carbohydrates. They were only half correct. It turns out that our brains actually crave calorically dense foods, which are foods loaded with sugar *and* fat. Make a short list of your favorite foods and chances are they contain both high levels of sugar and fat. Remember that insulin also stores fats as fat.

When it comes to protein, choose lean cuts of protein, and stick to monounsaturated or polyunsaturated fats. Eat as much as you like, at least initially. The first part of the SML diet is to get off the blood sugar rollercoaster and stop the binge eating.

Fats do not raise your blood sugar at all. Before you jump up and rejoice, be aware that saturated fats are unhealthy; they raise cholesterol levels and can cause heart and circulatory system damage.

Saturated fats come mainly from animal products like butter, cheese, and marbled meats such as steak. Therefore, try to minimize your consumption of saturated fat. The better forms of fat are monoun-saturated and polyunsaturated.

Monounsaturated fats are found in peanut and olive oils. Polyunsaturated fat is found in omega-3 fatty acids and canola oil. Canola or olive oil is often used in cooking sprays, but be sure to check the label. None of these fats harm your heart or circulatory system. In fact, consuming monounsaturated and polyunsaturated fats might even be beneficial. Although fat slows down the rate at which carbs enter into your bloodstream, their effect is small, so please don't add fat into your diet to slow down the carbs. While trying to break out of binge eating, fats can be eaten "to taste".

Protein is a weird nutrient. Protein never raises your blood sugar level. Certain types of protein can even lower your blood sugar by increasing the amount of insulin that is secreted. Most proteins, how-ever, don't do this, so it is best to stick to lean proteins. Avoid cuts of meat with marbled fat, and instead stick to meats such as turkey, chicken, low fat beef, some cuts of pork, and all fish.

USE YOUR NATURAL OFF SWITCH

We want to count and limit simple carbs, because we don't have a natural "off switch" telling us when to stop eating them. We do, however, have "off switches" for medium and long-acting carbs. Unfortunately, your greedy, sugar-loving brain doesn't naturally "stop" after you've eaten a "decent" amount of simple carbs (or an indecent amount for that matter). Instead, it will demand that you to keep going, keep eat-ing. "You can't eat just one!" is indeed truth in advertising!

You could "down" a 2000 calorie decadent dessert before the waiter notices that you want a coffee refill. If you instead try to con-sume 2000 calories of skim milk instead of the rich dessert, your cof-fee would become cold and your waiter would have left for the day. You simply can't eat that many calories of low or no-fat milk product at your meal without triggering your "off switch". Given 2000 calo-ries of non-starchy vegetables to eat, before you finish your meal, your waiter would not only be home, but he'd be fast asleep after watching a late movie. Finally, 2000 calories of meat or olive oil would produce rather nauseating results. The very thought makes most of us grimace. Bottom line: count and limit your simple carbs. Doing so will lead to weight loss and better control of your blood sugar level.

KEEP IT BALANCED

As a diabetic you have been encouraged to eat more frequently and in smaller amounts. No doubt we've all developed personal eating habits and schedules. Some of us stick to the traditional meal patterns of breakfast, lunch and dinner, while others of us no longer make a distinction. In many cases, our eating schedule is not totally our choice; it has to fit into the real world of work, family life, and other responsibilities. Therefore, for your new eating plan to work for you, your meal planning has to be individually tailored. Only you can do this, although a certified nutritionist can probably come up with ideas you've never considered.

Although the solution to diabetes weight loss is not about calorie counting, you might benefit from having a sense of how many calories you want to be in your daily diet, if for no other reason so that you can figure out how to *roughly* divide your meals. The amount of food you require depends on your gender, activity level, age, etc. Some of us ignore the advice to eat more frequently, and we continue to divide our daily food intake into three large meals. Some of us throw in one snack. Others of us will divide our intake into seven equal but small meals. We're all different. Once you know the general principles, and use some common sense, you are ready to roll. It is recommended that you:

1. Limit your simple carbs for the day. For snacks, you'll want to stick to around the 100 calories, and meals can go up to around the 200 calorie mark for simple carbs (that's 25-50 grams of simple carbs). This is the most important limitation, but you'll want to see how your favorite simple starches affect your blood sugar level. Avoiding spikes is the purpose of limiting simple carbs, but remember, simple carbs make you happy, so enjoy them in moderation.

2. On one hand, you want to feel free to eat an unlimited amount of medium carbs, because you have a natural shut off for

overconsumption. Remember they are limited to the no-fat or low fat milk and milk like products. Rather than thinking of them as a clump of assorted dairy products occupying a certain portion of the food on your plate (not that there is anything wrong with it if that is how you eat), you might discover that you are incorporating them into your meal in creative ways, to include enhancing the taste of vegetables. Once you get over the bingeing cycles, you might want to reconsider the "unlimited amount" suggestion and replacing it with a "reasonable amount" option. A dash of common sense goes a long way. Interestingly, few people have a problem with medium carb (milk) amounts or require a conscious effort to limit them, because they do have a natural shutoff. More often, we require occasional reminders to use them creatively because they benefit us by helping us feel full for a fairly long time. Some people try to conceptualize the "recommended" amount of medium-acting carbs as an amount equaling *approximately* the calories in the simple carbs consumed at that meal or snack. Give yourself some flexibility and let your glucose testing be your guide!

3.   When it comes to long-lasting carbs, eat to your heart's content! There is no way you are going to overeat long-lasting carbs. They'll help you feel full, and they'll release their carbs slowly. They are not loaded with calories, so there is no calorie limit, and one can't quite say how much space on your plate you want to devote to them. The only answer somewhat correct would be: "All the empty space." Just be mindful of the amount of other carbs or fats you find yourself using to make vegetables more palatable.

With some thought and effort, you'll have meals that are both satisfying and filling. Your meals will result in weight loss and they will also keep your blood sugar levels down. Your new lifestyle will begin with a conscious effort that requires some thoughtfulness, planning, and experimentation, such as trying new recipes covered in the next chapter. You'll find, however, that your meals are satisfying, and soon you'll slowly develop healthy eating habits. You'll be rewarded richly when you start shedding pounds. You may not start smiling at your vegetables, but you will certainly not grimace or snarl at them as often.

BLOOD GLUCOSE MONITORING

You'll want to monitor your blood sugar (glucose) level to learn how various SML carbs affect you. There is only one accurate way to know what is happening to your glucose level over time: measuring it with a blood glucose monitor. There is a wide variation among individuals in the degree to which their sugar levels rise with food. Whereas one person might find a 40 point rise after a slice of pizza, another diabetic's numbers might double that. Don't just pay attention to the numbers to ensure they are within an acceptable range. Pay close attention to how your blood sugar levels react to particular foods. Better yet, write them down. It pays to keep a running, written log of foods that seem to spike your blood glucose level. Writing things down helps preserve the memory even if you never go back to reread what you've written (although you are strongly encouraged to do so)! Over time, you will learn what simple carbs your body can handle and which simple carbs it cannot handle well.

It is ideal to measure your blood sugar level immediately before you eat a meal and one hour after. Measuring one hour after provides a rough estimate of your peak blood sugar level. It is often recommended to test two hours after a meal. This is equally valuable, but it often fails because we forget to test ourselves. Two hours after a meal, many of us have refocused our attention elsewhere. Some of us more forgetful souls use timers to remind us. Be it one hour or two hours, just be sure to test.

It is optimal to raise your blood sugar level no more than 40 points one hour after eating. Going from 100 to 120 mg/dl would be fantastic! Going from 100 to 220, however, might suggest a problem with your food choices. The 40-point rise is important, because if it goes up more than that in an hour, your body is probably releasing a lot of insulin to lower it.

It is also important to test your blood glucose at night before you go to bed and in the morning when you arise. Your morning glucose level, in most cases, provides you with your baseline for the day. If you fall below it, your body will consider your blood sugar level to be low, and it will react accordingly. "Low" in this case, is not the old standard definition of anything below 73 mg/dl. Your morning blood glucose level is also a nice measure of your overall progression. As your body fat decreases and your glucose levels stabilize, your morning blood glucose levels will be lower. Ultimately, it would be ideal to have it between 80 and 90 mg/dl. A hearty congratulation to you when you achieve this!

If you have a blood sugar spike, try walking it off. Exercise is pretty much the only way other than medication to counter elevated blood sugar levels. Within seconds of beginning your activity, your body will start to burn the sugar in your blood stream, and the amount of insulin released will decrease. However, if your blood sugar is extremely high (for example, over 350), exercise will not help and might even make matters worse. In addition, the insulin released during exercise becomes less resistant. In other words, exercise makes your insulin work better. Drinking water will not flush the excess sugar out of your system, as is sometimes believed. However, it might replace some of the water lost as your body tries to flush glucose out.

Dealing with Hypoglycemia

One important tip for the treatment of hypoglycemia (low blood sugar) is *not* to eat your favorite foods. Unfortunately, a hypoglycemic brain is impaired in its ability to think well, it wants immediate gratification and short-term goals reign. Long-term goals lose their voice and fade into the background. This makes for one ugly equation:

Short Term Thinking + Ravenous Appetite
+ Decadent Food = Binge Eating

You can avoid this situation by using glucose tablets. Unlike other common suggestions for treating hypoglycemia (such as consuming tasty sweets), we have a more neutral attitude towards glucose tablets. Getting to eat tasty treats to bring our glucose level up is like rewarding us for having low glucose levels. Our slow brain can't stop at just one either…oh no…we overdo it, and we start looking forward to our next hypoglycemic episode! Most of us will admit (some of us only under oath) to eating more decadent food than necessary to bring our blood sugar levels back to normal…hey, we're just being careful! The really honest among us will even admit we jump for joy knowing we have to bring our sugar level up. Once again, the old rumor mill has it that you have a special stash of your favorite sweet treats, "just in case". If you don't ditch them, you may be dancing with the devil…just trying to be helpful, you know.

A bigger advantage of glucose tablets is that they get your blood sugar up the quickest, faster than any other food source on earth… even your hidden stash! As soon as your sugar goes up, your brain stops the overwhelming craving, and you can once again think straight, which means being able to think beyond the "short-term goals only" mode. Once your long-term thinking abilities come back, you can make better food choices.

Although glucose tablets get your blood sugar up fast, they won't keep it there. Similar to throwing a life preserver to a troubled swimmer, it's a temporary measure that lasts five to fifteen minutes at most. It's then time to get something to eat within the normal parameters and get out of the danger zone.

Of course, it is better for us to prevent hypoglycemia than to treat it. You can do this by timing your meals and food intake along with your exercise plan. Put your knowledge of SML carbs to work.

KEEPING A FOOD DIARY

Now that you know how SML carbs affect your blood sugar level and appetite, and you know how to balance your meals and snacks with the best combination of SML carbs, you'll want to keep track of your food intake by starting a food diary. A food diary helps you learn how various foods affect your blood sugar and hunger levels. It is a simple log of what you eat and when you eat, and it is kept on a daily basis. We'll cover food diaries—the types and benefits of keeping one, etc.—in more detail a bit later. Before we start making our entries in the diary, however, we first want some delicious, healthy, satisfying meals and snacks to get our diary off to a good start. It is time to put theory into practice, so prepare to enter the SML kitchen!

✻   ✻   ✻

Chapter 6

PREPARE YOUR KITCHEN FOR SUCCESS

If you're wearing a "poufy" chef's hat in preparation for this chapter, you're probably overdressed. Although it's a thoughtful gesture on your part, you'll discover meal preparation according to the SML guidelines of *The Greenwich Diet*—eating the recommended balance of small, medium and long-acting carbs—isn't anywhere near as complex or involved as you might imagine. There is nothing radical about the SML meal planning. Although no special cooking skills are required, a little creativity on your part will serve you well. Because even your favorite old pair of shoes first required a bit of time to adjust for a comfortable fit, so too might your new SML meals. Eventually, however, the novelty will wear off and you'll be accustomed to your new approach to eating. You might find your transition to an SML balanced diet more inviting and even a bit easier if some of your apprehensions are put to rest. Here are some of the common misunderstandings voiced by one rather pessimistic person. Let's call her naysaying Norah:

MISUNDERSTANDINGS

1. "Good grief, I'll have to measure, weigh and count everything!"

   No you don't Norah. You'll want to keep track of what you eat by keeping a food diary, but most people lose weight without having to measure, weigh, or count anything. The only exception is limiting your intake of short-acting carbs—something you can easily do. Remember the short-acting carbs are sugar, white bread, etc.

2. "That's easy for you to say, but if I don't track calories or carbs, I won't lose weight!"

   Says who Norah? Actually, those of us who use common sense rather than a calculator seem to fare better. Strange, isn't it?

Perhaps this is because being constantly concerned with numbers creates a bit of a barrier or unnecessary challenge for many of us. Heck, we even try to pass the buck when it comes to calculating restaurant tips, so why would we want to engage in various forms of numerical measurements of our food? If you follow the SML diet recommendations and exercise, you will most likely lose weight. Only if you discover that you don't lose weight following this method will you want to reread the following chapter on accelerating weight-loss, which explores a calorie counting option including fun software apps. Most of us find our new lifestyle easier to embrace if we are not counting calories, carbs, points or ounces. Think of counting as a backup strategy.

3. "Yeah, sure, but didn't you just say that to lose weight I'll always need just the right balance of short, medium and long-acting carbs with each meal?"

Will you stop already Norah? There you are, talking about your "needs" again! Certainly, you "want" meals with a nice combination of SML carbs, but you don't always "need" them. Remember that you are transitioning to a new lifestyle, a better lifestyle, and perfectionism can derail your momentum. If you always expect perfection, you will experience failures. Failures can sabotage us. Let common sense be your guide. In the real world, missing a meal that doesn't have an ideal combination of carbs is going to happen. As long as you are headed in the right direction, you're going to get to your destination. The speed you choose to travel is up to you.

4. "I love food, and don't want to sacrifice my eating pleasure, darn it!"

Say what? Admittedly, this belief fools many of us; we simply can't imagine not having our favorite foods and also being able to walk away from a meal feeling satisfied. First, you don't have to give up your favorite foods; and second, Norah, you will walk away from an SML meal feeling satisfied. You may not want to eat *as much* of your favorites as you did in the past, but why not have a small portion? Many of us have found ways to modify our favorite foods to fit into the SML framework. Yes, it requires a bit of effort and creativity, but in most cases, it can be done.

5. "But I'm not a good cook!"

    So we've heard, but you don't have to possess great cooking skills to prepare SML meals. If you can put together a meal now, you can put together an SML meal. Further, there are many simple meals that can be made from prepared or semi-prepared foods that once "thrown together" make a satisfying SML meal. You can even dine out and stick to the SML guidelines if you order wisely and ask your waiter or waitress for substitutions when necessary.

6. "But my family probably won't eat my SML meals!"

    Do you really expect a hunger strike or perhaps another family petition against you? How your family responds is largely up to you. You'll have very few complaints if you choose dishes that you know your family will enjoy. You may have to look through a few more recipes and break away from the 10 meals you usually prepare or eat. Besides, remember you are not obligated to eat everything you prepare for the rest of your family. Just keep in mind it is hard…no… make that almost impossible to avoid eating certain foods when those foods are within reach. It is even more difficult when tempting aromas waft to your side of the dinner table, as they inevitably seem to do. Aromas elicit a primal urge to eat. You'll find if you don't make a big fuss with your family about your new way of eating, your family might not even notice the transition. Finally, SML meals are good for everyone, so there is no reason to feel guilty. Use it as an opportunity to establish good eating patterns in your family.

USEFUL TIPS

-   Plan your meals ahead of time. You can always make changes, but having a plan will help you stick to healthier practices. Unplanned, impromptu meals are often not well thought out and can take you off course. Here is a template for meal planning, but remember to allow yourself flexibility:

S-M-L Weekly Meal Plan

	Sunday	Monday	Tuesday	Wednesday	Thursday	Friday	Saturday
Breakfast							
Snack							
Lunch							
Snack							
Dinner							
Snack							

- Shop only for the meals you plan. Roaming through the store and buying "appealing" food items rather than those on your list makes meal preparation much more challenging. Further, having a stockpile of appealing foods calling your name from the refrigerator certainly doesn't help you stick to your long-term goals.

- Forget about being your county's coupon champion. Don't let coupons negatively influence your food selections. If they save you money on the foods already on your list, great! If they get you to select other foods not on your list, pass up the savings.

- Prepare foods that have more than one use. Multiuse foods such as dips and sauces can be used as dips for snacks, and sauces for meats and vegetables. Many can also be used as salad dressings.

- Search for diabetes-friendly meal recipes. Just be sure they limit the short-acting carbs (see below list) and add lots of veggies if needed.

- Many great diabetic-friendly meal recipes avoid or limit medium-acting carbs (low fat milk product group). Adding a "no sugar added" skim milk pudding or other no-fat dairy dessert, or a small glass of skim milk rounds out a meal nicely. Similarly, a bit of low or no-fat yogurt, sour cream or sprinkling of cheese is a handy and simple way of adding medium-acting carbs to meals that lack them.

- Think quantity. If you are going to take the time to cook a nice meal, make extra meals to freeze. If you plan ahead, this can be quite a time and money saver!

- Here's an old one worth repeating: Don't shop when you are hungry!

- Enjoy your favorite foods, and if necessary, give some thought to how you can adapt your favorites to better fit the SML framework. Broiling some thin strips of chicken breast and drenching them in a low-fat hot sauce might be a decent substitute for chicken wings. Enjoying pita chips made from low carb pita bread (such as Joseph's brand oat and flax pita) is a nice substitute for other types of salty snacks such as chips (recipe to follow).

- You can still enjoy some of your favorite food you fear will lead to overeating. The trick is to enjoy a smaller amount of them (buy only a small amount) and eat them at the end of your meal when you're close to being full. You'll be able to enjoy your favorites while lessening the temptation to overeat.

- When planning a meal, start with a concept such as "taco," "casserole," "stir fry," etc. You can then plan the ingredients you want to include in the dish. Hey, you've got to start somewhere!

- In some cases, you can eat your veggies and increase your portion size and sense of fullness by adding more non-starchy vegetables to common dishes. Finely chopped zucchini in a chili is almost undetectable; it adds volume and an extra vegetable. Chopped and boiled or sautéed cabbage, when well drained, along with green onions, can extend mashed potatoes as well as add flavor (a concoction not unlike Irish Colcannon potatoes). Bell peppers, of all colors, and mushrooms can be added to many dishes. "Throwing in" a few extra vegetables along the way allows you to continue to enjoy your favorite dishes and eat a healthy SML meal.

- When substituting a low-fat cheese in a recipe, the cheese might require a longer cooking time and a lower temperature to melt properly.

- Plan to use one grocery item more than once during the week. For example, Joseph's oat/flax pita can be used to make a pizza, a Greek rotisserie chicken sandwich with tzatziki sauce, etc. Dreamfields' pasta can be used in a hot dish such as Mac and Cheese and a cold pasta and vegetable salad a couple days later. Planning a week's worth of meals helps you select foods that do "double duty".

- Keep your shopping list visible and easily accessible. It helps your planning and eventual preparation much easier.

- Use "high speed" items to minimize preparation time. Items like frozen vegetables, lettuce mixes, precut vegetables, turkey meatballs, rotisserie chicken or packed pre-cooked chicken breast strips, salsas and bottled sauces, etc. are all time savers.

- Use the professional chef's approach of having all ingredients in place and ready before starting to prepare your meal. It increases efficiency and decreases the stress. Reading your recipe a few times before you start to cook will help prevent confusion, mistakes and the annoyance of having to double check.

- Eat more soups and add extra vegetables or a greater variety of vegetables to your favorite soups or stews.

- Adding some low-fat milk to broth-based soups increases the richness of many soups.

TRADE UP

Some of us look at our diet in such a new way it dawns on us there are recipes and food choices available that are better than the same limited number of meals we have come to rely upon out of habit. SML meals are hardly dramatic or extreme, and the meal options are almost endless. If you are willing (and able) to put in the time and effort to learn how to make new, adventurous meals, you may find the "tastiness" and "appeal" factors of your meals actually increase. You can, in effect, "trade up" from the way you have been eating. Handling and preparing food can be very satisfying for many of us, so here's a healthy challenge: Why not set one of your goals to "master" the art of SML meal preparation? Being able to prepare delicious and exciting SML meals can result in the satisfaction and pleasure that comes from mastery. The secret ingredients for mastering SML meal preparation skills are time and effort. If you put in enough time and effort, you can make and enjoy fabulous meals! Just be aware this approach, which requires a different type of focus on food, may not be suitable to some people. Some of us do best when our focus is on things other than food.

THE SHORT, MEDIUM AND LONG CARBS

Below you will find a list of short-, medium-, and long-acting carbs. Remember, you are going to limit your short-acting carbs, and it is highly unlikely you are going to overeat medium-acting carbs (low- or no-fat milk products or lentils), so you don't have to worry about eating too many of them. You will run into problems if you eat milk products that are not low fat or fat free. Feel free to eat long-acting carbs to your stomach's (and heart's) content.

The number of short-acting carbs you eat is best limited to a "normal" portion. A family size bag of potato chips is not a normal portion. Also, don't trust the number of carbs or calories in a "portion" on a food container without looking at the portion size to which they are referring. Most are unrealistic and even insulting. Remember, you want the satisfaction provided from eating short-acting carbs (we love that dopamine!) without spiking your blood sugar, so the "recommended" amount of short-acting carbs may vary somewhat between individuals. SML nutritionists usually avoid recommending we eat a specific number of the different types of carbs because they aren't individualized and numbers might distract and annoy us over the long-haul. Nevertheless, somewhere around 100 calories of simple carbs for snacks and 200 calories of simple carbs for meals are within the desired range. Please remember to be flexible and to let your hunger, weight and blood glucose tests be your guide.

SHORT-ACTING CARBOHYDRATES

Most of us with diabetes are expert in identifying short-acting (or simple) carbs. This does not stop food manufacturers and marketers from trying to convince us their food products comprise "complex carbohydrates" when in fact they are selling simple carbs. This is especially true when it comes to the plethora of whole grain or multigrain products. Although whole grain products take a bit longer to break down compared to simpler carbs such as sugar and refined white flour, and they are therefore preferred for that reason, the difference isn't anywhere near what the marketers suggest. Short-acting carbs include:

- Sugar: Yes, in all forms regardless of source, and this includes products that contain sugar such as honey, raw sugar, beet sugar, and corn syrup.

- Starchy vegetables: Potatoes, yams, corn, peas, legumes, and lima beans (except soy beans and lentils).

- Fruit and fruit juice: All fruit, but fruit naturally growing farther from the equator tends to have less sugar.

- Grains: All grains from wheat (regardless if they are whole, cracked or refined), rice, oats, corn, barley, etc.

- Cereals: Hey, they are made of grains, aren't they? We're still waiting for a good, tasty breakfast cereal…hint, hint you entrepreneurs!

EXAMPLES OF SNACK SIZE PORTIONS OF SHORT-ACTING CARBS

Here are some examples of suggested portions for short-acting carb snacks. You'll see some great ideas along with some paltry size portions for comparison:

- Most 100 calorie snack packs
- Bun top
- 1/4 of a bagel
- 1 slice of regular toast
- 1 light English muffin
- 2 slices of 40-45 calorie lite bread/toast
- 1 One Power brand Nut Natural bar
- 1 Kind brand bar
- 1 single serving 100 cal popcorn
- 1 cup Cheerios or cornflakes without milk
- 3/4 cup peas
- 1/3 cup of beans/ chick peas
- 4 tablespoons hummus
- 3/4 cup of whole corn

- 1 Joseph's Brand flax, oat & wheat pita, tortilla or lavash
- 3/4 hot dog bun
- 1 frozen waffle
- 1 small soft or hard taco shell
- 1 Balance brand bar: all flavors
- 1 Zone brand bar: all flavors
- 2 pretzel rods
- 6 Ritz crackers, plain
- 10 average potato chips
- 1 large apple with skin
- 1 cup diced pineapple
- 6 oz apple juice
- 4 oz orange juice
- 2 cups whole strawberries
- 1 + 1/4 cups blueberries

One of the most popular lines of snack products, because they are effective in controlling hunger, are Extend Nutrition brand bars, crisps, shakes and other product. Their doctor-developed nutrition products help control blood sugar levels up to 9 hours. Their website www.extendbar.com explains how their products work and where to buy them.

MEDIUM-ACTING CARBOHYDRATES

Cheeses

- Cheese slices: low-fat/fat-free
- Cottage cheese: low-fat/fat-free
- Feta cheese: reduced-fat
- Ricotta cheese: fat-free/low-fat
- Cheeses: fat-free/low fat varieties, e.g. 2 oz. Cabot's 75% fat-free
- Soft cheese: Laughing Cow brand low-fat cheese
- Low-fat cheese sticks

Milks

- Evaporated skim, fat-free/low-fat
- Skim milk

Cultured Milk Products

- Buttermilk
- Buttermilk: fat-free/low-fat
- Buttermilk: non-fat dry
- Greek yogurt: non-fat/no fat plain Greek yogurt
- Kefir: non-fat plain
- Milk: non-fat dry
- Sour cream: non-fat/fat-free varieties
- Yogurt: non-fat/fat free without added sugar

Sweets

- Chocolate drink: no sugar added Swiss Miss brand hot chocolate
- Frozen yogurts: low-fat/non-fat, no sugar added
- Ice cream: low-fat/no-fat, no sugar added ice cream (Edie's brand has one, also Slim-a-Bear brand products)
- Pops: Weight Watcher's brand pops
- Pudding: sugar-free brands, e.g. Cozy Shack brand no sugar added

Soy Products

- Soy beans (aka Edamame)
- Soy cheese
- Soy milk: unflavored
- Tofu

Other

- Dreamfields brand pasta
- Lentils

LONG-ACTING CARBOHYDRATES

- Amaranth (Chinese spinach)
- Artichoke
- Artichoke hearts
- Asparagus
- Baby corn
- Bamboo shoots
- Bean sprouts
- Broccoli (which when eaten with a sufficient amount of tomato product is the only vegetable associated with a lower rate of prostate cancer!)
- Brussels sprouts (try shredding and sautéing if you are not a fan.)
- Cabbage: green, Chinese, bok choy,
- Beans: green, wax, Italian
- Beets
- Carrots (but don't throw away your glasses just yet!)
- Cauliflower
- Celery
- Chayote
- Cucumber
- Daikon radish
- Eggplant
- Gourds: delicate, gooseneck, etc.
- Green onions (scallions)
- Greens: collard, kale, mustard, turnip
- Hearts of palm
- Jicama
- Kohlrabi
- Lettuce: all varieties
- Leeks
- Mung bean sprouts
- Mushrooms: all fresh varieties
- Okra (stir frying in hot oil helps prevent slime.)
- Onions
- Pea pods
- Peppers: all varieties
- Pickles: bread and butter (no-sugar added), dill
- Pumpkin
- Radishes

- Rutabaga
- Salad greens
- Sauerkraut
- Soybean sprouts
- Spinach
- Squash (all types)
- Sugar snap peas
- Swiss chard
- Tomato
- Turnips
- Water chestnuts
- Yard-long beans

TIPS FOR ENHANCING VEGETABLES

Variety is the spice of life, and your vegetables can become more attractive if you add variety. Here are some tips:

1. Search your grocery store for vegetables you are not accustomed to buying or eating. Many of us stick to the same 5 or 6 vegetables, whereas many more are available if we look both in the fresh and frozen food sections.

2. Vegetables can taste quite differently depending on their cooking method. Vary the way you prepare your vegetables. Here are some options:

   - Stir fry with a small amount of oil; add herbs and/or spices, garlic or fresh ginger.
   - Grill either outdoors or indoors with a grill pan.
   - Broil. A quick spray of cooking oil assists browning and helps the spices to adhere. Rotate half way through broiling. If using a variety of vegetables, cut them to size so they are all done at the same time.
   - Steam.
   - Cream (okay, puree) them into a soup (recipe below).

3. Try raw or blanched vegetables with a low-fat dip.

4. Spice them up with…well…spices! There are many spice mixes available in the spice section of your store, or you can easily make your own concoction. Explore spices with which you are less familiar. There's now a whole new tasty world of spices available that your grandmother would never recognize. Fresh herbs, although somewhat expensive, can provide incredible flavor and appeal. A fresh squeeze of lemon or lime can also enhance their appeal. True brand powdered lemon, lime and orange, in single serve, non-perishable packets, according to many, are as tasty as the real thing. Garlic, of course, gives vegetables sex appeal as well as wards off vampires.

5. Add flavor to your veggies by topping them with a dollop of sauce or cheese. Just be sure to use the low fat types.

6. There is hardly a dish to which you can't sneak in a few vegetables, from a simple burger to a casserole.

FOODS TO ADD "MEAL APPEAL" BUT NOT USED AS A BASE FOR A MEAL

- Chicken
- Lean beef
- Ham (lean)
- Canadian bacon
- All fish
- Olivio brand products
- Low-fat turkey products (e.g., turkey bacon)

- All shellfish
- Olive oil
- Vegetable sprays
- Canola oil
- Smart Balance
- No fat/low-fat hot dogs

PROBLEMATIC FOODS

Some popular foods are extremely difficult to eat in reasonable portions. Your brain will be insulted by the meager serving and demand more! Here are just some of them:

- Bagel
- Pizza—deep dish or Sicilian style
- Panini sandwiches
- Chips—baked, regular, potato or corn
- Cereal
- Wraps or burritos (the high calories ones)

- Pita (regular ones)
- Muffins
- Scones
- Cake
- Cookies

SMALL PORTION FOOD

Due to their high saturated fat content, limit your portions of the following foods to very small portions, perhaps a teaspoon at the most.

- Butter
- Ice cream
- Regular cheese
- Foie gras
- Liver
- Liverwurst
- Pepperoni

- Cream
- Bacon
- Hot Dog
- Non chicken or turkey sausages
- Full fat beef
- Balogna
- Salami

MENUS AND RECIPES

You don't require special recipes to cook SML meals. Many of your favorite recipes and meals can be modified to fit your SML meal plan. If you think of a meal on your plate as consisting of portions of proteins, fats, short-acting carbs, medium-acting carbs, and long-acting carbs, the SML way of eating is nothing more than adjusting the portions of each. But just because SML meal planning and preparation isn't difficult, doesn't mean we can't appreciate some good recipes and short-cuts.

☆   ☆   ☆

Chapter 7

DELICIOUS AND SATISFYING RECIPES

Breakfast commonly consists of short-acting carbs such as grains in cereals or things like bacon, eggs, potatoes, or fruit. You'd be hard-pressed to name your favorite breakfast vegetable, but you won't have to if you prepare one of the following single-serving SML breakfasts:

Scram-wich

1 x 100% whole wheat English muffin
1 whole egg plus1 egg white
Salt and pepper to taste
1/3 cup frozen spinach, thawed, drained
1/4 cup reduced-fat cheddar cheese
1 slice fresh tomato
1 ounce thinly sliced low-sodium cooked ham or Canadian bacon

Preparation:

1. In a small bowl, whisk eggs with salt and pepper to taste.

2. Lightly spray an unheated, non-stick 6" skillet with cooking spray. Heat skillet over medium heat.

3. Add eggs and cook, stirring often until eggs are almost set.

4. Toast a split English muffin.

5. Add spinach and cheese to egg and continue to cook for approximately 2 more minutes (until spinach warms, cheese melts, and eggs set).

6. Place ham, tomato, and scrambled egg mixture on one half of muffin. Add additional salt and pepper to taste. Top with other muffin half. Enjoy, but smile in the mirror after eating to check your teeth for spinach!

Veggie Omelet

1 slice 100% whole grain bread
1 whole egg plus 2 egg whites
Salt and pepper to taste
1/4 cup tomatoes, diced
1/4 cup yellow onion, diced
1/4 cup green onion, chopped
1/4 cup bell pepper, diced
1/4 cup button mushrooms, sliced
1/4 cup reduced-fat or part-skim shredded mozzarella cheese
1 teaspoon grated Romano cheese

Preparation:

1. In a small bowl, whisk eggs and add salt and pepper to taste.

2. Lightly spray an unheated, non-stick 6" skillet with cooking spray. Heat skillet over medium heat.

3. Add onion, pepper, and mushrooms. Cook until slightly softened, about 2 minutes. Add tomato and green onion and cook for another minute.

4. Toast bread slice.

5. Add eggs to the sautéed vegetables and allow them to spread over entire skillet. Cook until eggs are almost set.

6. Sprinkle the mozzarella and Romano cheeses over eggs. Place spatula under one edge of eggs and fold over before removing from pan.

7. Add additional salt and pepper to taste. Serve with toast.

Wake-up Wrap

1 x 6" soft whole wheat tortilla
1 whole egg plus 1 egg white
Salt and pepper to taste
2 ounces skinless, cooked chicken breast, diced
2 tablespoons shredded, reduced-fat Mexican blend cheese
3 tablespoons all-natural, vegetable salsa
1 tablespoon fat-free sour cream

Preparation:

1. In a small microwave proof bowl, whisk the eggs and add salt and pepper to taste. Add the chicken.

2. Microwave for about 2 minutes or until the eggs have set and chicken is warmed through.

3. Layer the cooked eggs, cheese, sour cream, and salsa onto the tortilla.

4. Fold tortilla over and serve.

Steak & Eggs Pizza

1 Joseph's brand oat and flax low-carb pita
1/4 cup all-natural, no sugar added, prepared tomato sauce
1 whole egg plus 1 egg white
Salt and pepper to taste
2 ounces thinly sliced, cooked lean steak
1 cup mixed bell peppers, sliced
1/4 cup yellow onion, sliced
1/2 cup button mushrooms, sliced
2 slices reduced-fat white cheese slices

Preparation:

1. Preheat oven to 400F. In a small bowl, whisk eggs and add salt and pepper to taste.

2. Lightly spray an unheated, non-stick 6" skillet with cooking spray. Heat skillet over medium heat.

3. Add onion, pepper, and mushrooms and cook until slightly softened (about 3 minutes).

4. Spread tomato sauce over top of pita. Top with eggs, sliced steak, peppers, onions, and mushrooms.

5. Lay cheese slices over top of filled pita.

6. Place pita in oven directly on middle rack and cook for 8-10 minutes. When desired crispness is achieved, carefully remove pizza from oven. Cut into four pieces.

Breakfast Tostada

1 cup baked corn tortilla chips
1 whole egg plus 1egg white
Salt and pepper to taste
1 ½ cups romaine lettuce, chopped
1/2 cup tomato, chopped
1/2 cup bell pepper, chopped
1/4 green onion (scallion)
1/4 cup sliced canned black olives, drained, rinsed
1/4 cup canned black beans, drained, rinsed
1/4 cup shredded, reduced-fat Mexican cheese blend
3 tablespoons all-natural vegetable salsa
1 tablespoon fat-free sour cream

Preparation:
1. In a small microwave safe bowl, whisk the eggs, black beans, and add salt and pepper to taste.

2. Microwave the egg-bean mixture for about 2 minutes or until the eggs have set and black beans are warmed through.

3. Place chips on serving plate spreading into a single layer. Break up the cooked eggs-bean mixture and layer over the chips.

4. Top with cheese, lettuce, tomato, bell pepper, green onion, and black olives.

5. Garnish with salsa and sour cream.

Mini Bagel and Veggie Cream Cheese

1 x 100% whole wheat mini bagel
1/2 cup vegetable cream cheese (recipe below)

Preparation:
1. Toast mini bagel to desired doneness.

2. Top each bagel half with 1/4 cup cream cheese mix

Vegetable Cream Cheese

1 x 8 ounce container fat-free cream cheese
1/4 cup green onion, finely chopped
1/4 cup red bell pepper, seeded, small diced
1/4 cup radish, finely diced
1/4 cup carrot, finely diced
1/4 cup celery, small diced
1/4 cup cucumber, seeded, small diced
Salt and pepper to taste

Preparation:
1. Place cream cheese in a medium bowl. Add all remaining ingredients and fold the remaining ingredients into the cream cheese with a rubber spatula until thoroughly combined.

2. Cover with plastic wrap and refrigerate until needed.

Cherry Tomato-Broccoli Frittata

1 whole egg plus 1 egg white
Salt and pepper to taste
1 teaspoon extra virgin olive oil
1/2 cup frozen chopped broccoli, thawed
1/2 cup yellow onion, small diced
1/2 cup cherry tomatoes, quartered
2 tablespoons reduced-fat feta cheese

Preparation:
1. Preheat broiler. In a small bowl, whisk eggs with salt and pepper to taste. Stir in cheese.

2. Heat oil in small broiler-proof skillet over medium heat. Cook broccoli and onion until warmed and tender, about 3 minutes.

3. Pour egg mixture over broccoli mixture in skillet,

4. Reduce heat to medium low. As eggs cook, occasionally run a rubber spatula around the edge of the skillet, lifting egg mixture so uncooked portion flows underneath. When almost set, place tomatoes on top of egg mixture.

5. Place skillet under the broiler about 4-5" inches from the heat for about 3-4 minutes or until center sets completely. Cut into four wedges.

SNACK AND LIGHT MEAL IDEAS

Call these versatile recipes anything you want: snacks, smacks, light meals, munchies, appetizers…they are all good!

Joseph's Pita Chips

Joseph's Brand flax, oat, and whole wheat pitas
Vegetable spray (olive oil preferred)
Salt
Spices (optional): onion powder, garlic powder, or curry powder.

Preparation:
1. Separate pitas to get two ovals from each pita. Cut or tear them into bite size pieces.

2. Cover baking tray with foil and lightly coat with vegetable spray.

3. Place pita pieces on tray and lightly spray again with vegetable spray.

4. Sprinkle the pieces with salt and desired spices.

5. Bake at 350F degrees for about 5 minutes or until slightly brown. Watch carefully, because they burn quickly. Nice with a dip!

Roasted Garbanzo Beans (Chickpeas)

1 x 15-oz or 19-oz can of garbanzo beans
Cooking oil spray or 1 tablespoon olive oil
Salt
Garlic powder (optional)
Onion powder (optional)
Cayenne pepper (optional and use sparingly) or curry powder

Preparation:
1. Preheat oven to 400F degrees

2. Drain and dry garbanzos with paper towel.

3. Toss beans in a bowl with spices and coat with cooking spray or 1 tablespoon of olive oil.

4. Spread evenly on a baking sheet covered with aluminum foil and bake on middle rack until crunchy, about 30 minutes.

Spicy Buffalo Legs
Servings: 4 (4 pieces of celery + 1/4 cup no-fat or low-fat cream cheese spread)

4 celery ribs, trimmed and cut into 3"-long pieces (16 pieces total)
1 cup fat-free cream cheese
8 teaspoons Frank's hot sauce,
1/4 cup crumbled blue cheese
1 teaspoon fresh ground black pepper
1/4 teaspoon fresh lemon juice

Preparation:
1. In a small bowl, mix cream cheese, hot sauce, blue cheese, and black pepper until combined.

2. Spread the cream cheese mixture into the channel portion of each piece of celery.

Cheese Steak Rollups with Boursin Cheese, Mushrooms, Peppers and Onions
Servings: 4 (each portion is 4 rollups)

16 (about 8 ounces) slices of cooked beef, such as tenderloin or fresh deli roast beef
1 cup lite Boursin cheese, softened
2 ½ tablespoons steak sauce
3 ounces red, yellow, orange, and/or green bell peppers, seeded
2 ounces red onion, peeled, thinly sliced
3 ounces cooked whole Portobello mushroom caps, thinly sliced

Preparation:

1. Spread each steak slice with 1 teaspoon Boursin cheese.

2. Top with bell peppers, onion, and mushrooms.

3. Drizzle equal amount of steak sauce on each.

4. Roll the steak around the bell pepper slices.

Loaded "Baked" Potato
Servings: 2

2 medium Yukon Gold potatoes
1/4 cup frozen broccoli, thawed, chopped
1/4 cup frozen spinach, thawed, drained, chopped
1/4 cup roasted red peppers, drained, rinsed, chopped
1/4 cup scallion, thinly sliced
1/4 cup red onion, peeled, diced
1/4 cup artichoke hearts, drained, rinsed, chopped
2 bacon strips, cooked, drained, chopped
1/2 cup reduced-fat cheddar cheese
2 tablespoons fat-free feta cheese
2 tablespoons fat-free sour cream
1/2 cup all-natural, no-sugar added, vegetable salsa

Preparation

1. Take a fork and poke holes in the potatoes.

2. Place in the microwave and cook according to your micro-waves specifications, about 10-12 minutes or until potatoes are soft through the middle.

3. Place on a plate and cut potatoes halfway down the middle and fold open.

4. In a separate medium-size bowl, mix broccoli, spinach, red peppers, scallions, red onion, artichoke hearts, feta cheese, and bacon until combined, and top each potato with half the mixture.

5. Sprinkle each potato with cheddar cheese and return to the microwave. Cook on high for 1 minute or until ingredients are warm and cheese is melted.

6. Top each potato with sour cream and salsa.

Petite Salad Pizza
Servings: 1

1 x 100% whole wheat English muffin
2 tablespoons all-natural, no-sugar added, tomato sauce
2 tablespoons part-skim, reduced-fat shredded mozzarella cheese
1 cup spring mix lettuces
1/4 cup carrot, shredded
1/4 cup cucumber, seeded, quartered, sliced
2 teaspoons red wine vinegar
1 teaspoon extra virgin olive oil
Salt and black pepper to taste

Preparation:
1. Preheat oven to 400F.

2. Split English muffin and place both halves ridged side up on flat surface.

3. Spread 1 tablespoon tomato sauce on each half and top each with 1 tablespoon of shredded mozzarella cheese.

4. Bake in oven directly on wire rack for about 8-10 minutes.

5. While pizza is baking, in a small bowl mix spring mix, carrots, cucumber, vinegar, olive oil, salt, and pepper until coated.

6. Remove English muffin pizza from the oven and top each half with salad.

Four Corners Quesadilla
Servings: 1

1 x 6" lower-carb tortilla per serving
1 tablespoon soft chevre (goat) cheese, crumbled
1/4 cup reduced-fat shredded Mexican blend cheese
2 ounces cooked rotisserie chicken
1/2 cup frozen chopped spinach, thawed, drained
1/4 cup canned, diced green chilies, rinsed, drained

2 tablespoons prepared all-natural vegetable salsa
1 tablespoon fat-free sour cream

Preparation
1. Place tortilla on a flat surface. Spread shredded cheese, crumbled cheese, green chilies, and spinach evenly over one side of the tortilla. Place cooked chicken on top.

2. Fold the empty side of the tortilla over onto the other side that has the ingredients to make a half moon shape.

3. Preheat a medium-sized sauté pan over medium heat, and spray lightly with cooking spray. Place the quesadilla onto the pan and cook one side until lightly browned and crisp, about 4 minutes. Carefully flip the quesadilla over with a spatula and cook another 4 minutes or until other side is lightly browned and crisp.

4. Remove quesadilla from the pan. Cut into 2-3 wedges, and top with sour cream and salsa.

Green Eggs & Ham on Crackers
Servings: 1

2 large hard-boiled eggs, yolks discarded, chopped
1/2 cup fresh baby spinach, washed, chopped
1 tablespoon unsweetened pickle relish
2 teaspoons reduced-fat mayonnaise
2 teaspoons fat-free Greek yogurt
1/2 teaspoon Dijon mustard
1 slice (1-ounce) low-fat cooked ham, chopped
4 whole wheat saltine crackers

Preparation:
1. Place mayonnaise, yogurt, Dijon mustard, salt, and black pepper in a small bowl and whisk to combine.

2. Fold in hard egg whites, baby spinach, ham and mix to combine.

3. Spread mixture among 4 crackers.

Quickie Kabobs with Creamy Balsamic Vinaigrette
Servings: 4 (2 skewers and 1/4 cup creamy balsamic vinaigrette)

8 x 6" bamboo skewers
8 bocconcini mozzarella balls (the small ones)
8 cherry tomatoes
1 small yellow squash
1 small zucchini, cut into 8 x 1" pieces
4 slices of low-fat smoked deli chicken breast, halved
1 small cucumber, halved, seeded, cut into 8 x 1 inch pieces
1 red bell pepper, seeded, stemmed, cut into 8 pieces
1/2 cup fat-free plain Greek yogurt
1/4 cup balsamic vinegar
1/4 cup extra virgin olive oil
Salt and pepper to taste

Preparation:
1. Place on each skewer: 1 mozzarella ball, 1 cherry tomato, 1 piece each yellow and zucchini squashes, 1/2 slice chicken breast folded, 1 piece cucumber, and 1 piece red bell pepper.

2. In a small bowl, whisk together yogurt, balsamic vinegar, olive oil, salt and pepper until combined. Serve with kabobs.

Artichoke and Baby Spinach Spread with Sun-dried Tomatoes on Rubschlager Brand Mini Rye
Servings: 4 (4 slices of rye + 4 tablespoons spread each)

1 x 8 ounce package reduced-fat cream cheese
1/4 cup lite mayonnaise
1/4 cup grated Romano cheese
1/4 cup yellow onion, minced
1 clove garlic, minced
1/2 teaspoon dry basil
1/2 teaspoon dry oregano
1 x 14-ounce can artichoke hearts, drained, rinsed
1 cup frozen, chopped spinach, thawed, drained
1/2 cup sun-dried tomato
1/4 cup shredded, part-skim, reduced-fat mozzarella cheese
Salt and pepper to taste

Preparation:

1. Preheat oven to 350F.

2. Lightly spray a small baking dish with cooking spray.

3. In a medium bowl, mix together the cream cheese, mayonnaise, Romano cheese, onion, garlic, sun-dried tomatoes, salt, pepper, basil, and oregano.

4. Gently fold in the spinach and artichoke hearts.

5. Transfer the mixture to the prepared baking dish. Top with mozzarella cheese. Bake in the oven for about 25 minutes or until hot and bubbly.

6. Serve warm or cold.

SALADS AND SALAD DRESSINGS

Turkey BLT Salad with Buttermilk Dressing
Servings: 2

Salad
4 cups Romaine lettuce, washed and chopped
8 ounces sliced, cooked turkey
4 strips cooked bacon, drained, patted
1 cup pear or cherry tomatoes, halved
1/2 cup green onion/scallion, thinly sliced
2 pieces 100% whole wheat bread, toasted, cubed

Dressing
2 tablespoons lite mayonnaise
1/3 cup low-fat buttermilk
2 tablespoons apple cider vinegar
1 tablespoon extra virgin olive oil
1/4 cup fresh basil, chopped
Salt and black pepper to taste

Preparation:

1. To make dressing, place yogurt and remainder of dressing ingredients in a small bowl and whisk to combine.

2. To make salad, combine all salad ingredients and cubed toast in a medium bowl. Top with dressing and toss to coat salad.

Buffalo Grilled Shrimp Salad with Creamy Blue Cheese Dressing
Servings: 2

<u>Salad</u>
4 cups romaine lettuce, chopped
8 ounces frozen, cooked, peeled, and deveined shrimp, thawed
1/4 cup red hot sauce
1 cup, celery, washed, sliced thinly on the bias
1/2 cup red onion, thinly sliced
1/2 cup shredded carrots
1/2 cup green bell pepper
1/2 cup red bell pepper
1/2 cup cucumber, washed, halved, seeded, sliced

<u>Dressing</u>
1/4 cup fat-free plain Greek yogurt
1/4 cup lite mayonnaise
1 tablespoon lemon juice
1/8 teaspoon cracked black pepper
3 tablespoons fat-free milk
1 tablespoon blue cheese

Preparation:
1. To make dressing, combine all dressing ingredients in a small bowl and whisk to combine. Refrigerate until needed.

2. In a small bowl add thawed shrimp and hot sauce. Toss to coat.

3. Coat an unheated grill pan with cooking spray. Preheat grill pan over medium high heat.

4. Place shrimp on grill pan and cook for 3-5 minutes or until grill marks appear on the shrimp. Flip the shrimp over and repeat on the other side.

5. To make the salad, place salad ingredients in a medium bowl. Add shrimp and dressing. Toss to coat.

Smoked Salmon-Bacon Cobb Salad with Lemon-Caper Dressing
Servings: 2

Salad
6 ounces smoked salmon lox
2 hard egg whites, chopped
1 cup cherry tomatoes, halved
1/2 cup red onion, diced
1 cup cucumber, seeded, peeled, diced
1/2 avocado, peeled, seeded, diced
2 x 100% whole wheat mini bagels, toasted or 1 cup plain bagel chips

Dressing
8 ounces fat-free Greek yogurt
1/2 cup capers, drained, chopped
1/4 cup fresh lemon juice
1 teaspoon fresh lemon zest
1 tablespoon dry dill
Salt and black pepper to taste

Preparation:
1. To make dressing, combine all dressing ingredients in a small bowl and whisk until combined. Refrigerate until ready to use.

2. Heat a non-stick skillet over medium heat. Place smoked salmon flat on pan and cook until crisp. Flip and repeat on other side. Remove from heat and place on a paper towel to drain.

3. To make the salad, combine all salad ingredients except salmon, in a medium bowl. Toss with dressing to coat. Place salmon-bacon on top.

Warm Herbed Roasted Chicken Salad with Creamy Lemon-Garlic Vinaigrette
Servings: 2

Salad
2 teaspoons extra virgin olive oil
8 ounces boneless, skinless chicken breast
1/4 cup mixed fresh herbs, chopped (parsley, sage, rosemary, thyme)

4 cups spring salad mix
1 bunch asparagus, trimmed of thick stem
4 fresh garlic cloves, peeled
4 small red bliss potatoes, quartered
1 small onion, peeled, quartered
1 cup Crimini mushrooms, quartered
1 medium ripe tomato, chopped
Salt and black pepper to taste

<u>Dressing</u>
2 tablespoons fresh lemon juice
1 tablespoon lite mayonnaise
2 tablespoons non-fat, plain Greek yogurt
Salt and pepper to taste

Preparation:

1. Preheat oven to 375F.

2. In a small bowl, toss uncooked chicken breast with 1 teaspoon olive oil, fresh herbs, salt, and pepper to coat. Place on a cookie tray.

3. In another medium bowl, toss potatoes, garlic cloves, mushrooms, and asparagus with the remainder 1 teaspoon of oil. Place potatoes on a cookie tray.

4. Place cookie tray with chicken, garlic, onions, mushrooms, and potatoes in the oven and bake until the chicken is thoroughly cooked through (180 degrees internal temp/juices run clear) and potatoes are fork tender. This takes approximately 20 minutes.

5. About 10 minutes into the cooking, add asparagus to the oven tray.

6. Remove the tray when all ingredients are cooked. Allow to cool for 5 minutes.

7. To make dressing, remove roasted garlic from tray and place in a small bowl with the remainder of the dressing ingredients and whisk to combine. Set aside until needed.

8. To make the salad, slice chicken and asparagus, and place in a medium bowl with spring mix, mushrooms, onions, and potatoes. Toss with dressing to coat.

Crispy Chicken Cordon Bleu Salad with Honey and Grain Mustard Dressing
Servings: 2

<u>Salad</u>
4 cups baby spinach, washed and dried
4 breaded chicken tenderloin strips, cooked, chopped
2 slices low-fat Swiss cheese, chopped
2 ounces low-fat cooked ham, chopped
1 cup cherry tomatoes, halved
1/2 cup Bermuda red onion, peeled, sliced
1 cup cucumbers, quartered, seeded, chopped

<u>Dressing</u>
1 tablespoon honey
1 tablespoon Dijon mustard
3 tablespoons white wine vinegar
1 tablespoon extra virgin olive oil
2 tablespoons fat-free Greek yogurt
1 clove fresh garlic, minced

Preparation:
1. Cook chicken tenders according to manufacturer's suggestions until fully cooked. Remove from oven and set aside

2. To make the dressing, place all dressing ingredients in a small bowl and whisk to combine.

3. To make salad, combine all salad ingredients in a medium bowl and toss with dressing to coat.

Semi-Caesar Salad with Balsamic-Chevre (Goat Cheese) Dressing
Servings: 2

<u>Salad</u>
4 cups romaine lettuce
1 cup seasoned croutons

8 ounces boneless, skinless, chicken breast, cooked
1 cup cucumber, halved, seeded, sliced
1/2 cup sun-dried tomatoes, rehydrated
1 tablespoon goat cheese crumbles
1/2 cup mandarin orange segments, drained, rinsed
1/4 cup scallion, thinly sliced
1 tablespoon walnuts, chopped

<u>Dressing</u>
1 ½ tablespoons balsamic vinegar
1 ½ tablespoons lemon juice
1/2 teaspoon Dijon mustard
1 tablespoon lite mayonnaise
2 tablespoons fat-free Greek yogurt
1 tablespoon goat cheese crumbles
Black pepper to taste

Preparation:
1. To make dressing, combine all dressing ingredients in a small bowl and whisk to combine.

2. To make the salad, place all salad ingredients in a medium bowl and toss with dressing to coat.

Everything But the Kitchen Sink Salad with Simple Vinaigrette
Servings: 2

<u>Salad</u>
4 cups of any kind of lettuce, chopped
2 cups of fresh, frozen, roasted, grilled, raw, or blanched vegetables
8 ounces of cooked lean protein, whatever is available
1/2 cup shredded, sliced, or crumbled low-fat cheese (whatever is available)

<u>Dressing</u>
1/4 cup of any kind of vinegar
2 tablespoons olive oil, canola, or vegetable oil
1 tablespoon whatever fresh or dried herbs and spices you prefer and are available

Preparation:
1. To make the dressing, place all dressing ingredients in a small bowl and whisk to combine.

2. To make the salad, toss all salad ingredients in a medium bowl and toss with dressing to coat.

SOUPS

Soups are an ideal way of working lots of vegetables into meals. Feel free to mix and match your vegetables and come up with your own soup!

Basic Faux (Fake) Cream of Vegetable Soup

Your choice or combination of vegetables: zucchini, broccoli (or both), butternut squash, etc.
1 tablespoon olive oil
Onion (one small per quart of soup)
Chicken or vegetable broth or stock, enough to cover vegetables
Salt and pepper to taste
Choice of spice: Dried thyme, dill, or curry powder, etc.
Skim milk
Greek no-fat yogurt (optional)

Preparation:
1. Dice and sauté onion in soup pot until just starting to brown.

2. Chop vegetables into bite-sized pieces and place into pot and stir.

3. Cover vegetables and onion with just enough broth to just cover the vegetables.

4. Add salt, pepper and preferred spice(s) to taste and simmer until soft (about 20 minutes).

5. Puree vegetables and broth in blender or turn off the heat and use an immersion blender to puree vegetables and stock in the pot. Return to pot if you used blender.

6. Add skim milk to lighten appearance, about 1/4 cup per soup bowl serving. Taste and adjust spices.

7. Serve hot or cold with a dollop of low-fat yogurt or sour cream (or blend it in). Cold, it is a great snack and easily stored in a pitcher after it is cooled.

Broccoli-Cheddar Chowder
Servings: 6 (1 cup per serving)

1 tablespoon extra virgin olive oil
1 large onion, chopped
1 large carrot, diced,
2 stalks celery, diced
1 medium potato, peeled, and diced
2 cloves garlic, peeled and diced
1 tablespoon all-purpose flour
1/2 teaspoon dry mustard
1/8 teaspoon cayenne pepper,
28 ounces vegetable or chicken broth
8 ounces broccoli florets cut into small pieces
1 cup reduced-fat cheddar cheese
1/2 cup fat-free sour cream
Salt and pepper to taste

Preparation:
1. Heat olive oil in a large saucepan over medium-high heat. Add the onion, carrot, and celery and cook until the onion and celery are softened, stirring frequently, about 6 minutes.

2. Add the potato and garlic. Cook stirring often for another 2 minutes.

3. Stir in the flour, dry mustard and cayenne pepper. Cook stirring frequently for another 2 minutes.

4. Add the broth and broccoli stems and bring to a boil. Cover and reduce the heat to medium. Simmer, stirring occasionally, for about ten minutes. Stir in the florets and simmer, covered, until the broccoli is tender, about 8 more minutes.

5. Transfer about 2 cups of the chowder to a bowl and mash. Return to the pot.

6. Stir in the cheddar and sour cream. Cook over medium heat, stirring, until the cheese is melted and the chowder is heated through, about 2 more minutes. Season with salt and pepper to taste.

Lentil-Vegetable Soup
Servings: 6 (1 cup soup + 2 tablespoons of cheese per serving)

1 ½ tablespoons olive oil
1 + 1/3 cups diced onion
1/3 cup diced celery
1/3 cup diced carrot
2 bay leaves
2 tablespoons no-sugar-added tomato paste
1 teaspoon salt
2 garlic cloves, minced
6 cups fat-free, low-sodium vegetable or chicken stock
1 x 15-ounce can no-added-salt diced tomatoes,
1 cup dried French dark green or other lentils such as brown
1 block frozen chopped spinach (9 or 10 oz), thawed
1/3 cup chopped, fresh parsley
2 teaspoons red wine vinegar
2 teaspoons Dijon mustard
1/4 teaspoon black pepper
3/4 cup (3 ounces) shaved fresh Parmesan cheese

Preparation:
1. Heat the olive oil in a large saucepan over medium-high heat.

2. Add the diced onion, celery, carrot, and bay leaves. Sauté for about 8 minutes.

3. Add the tomato paste, salt, and minced garlic. Sauté 1 minute longer.

4. Add 6 cups stock, tomatoes, and lentils. Bring mixture to a boil, partially covered, and reduce heat and simmer the mixture for about 25 minutes.

5. Stir in the chopped spinach, parsley, vinegar, mustard and pepper. Cook 10 minutes.

6. Discard the bay leaves. Sprinkle with cheese before serving.

Corn, Bell Pepper, and Tomato Chowder
Servings: 6 (1 ½ cups + 2 teaspoons cheese + 1 teaspoon chives per serving)

3 red bell peppers, halved, seeded
2 cups frozen corn,
1 ½ pounds tomatoes, halved
1 tablespoon extra virgin olive oil
1/2 cup scallion/green onion, sliced thinly
4 cups yellow onion, chopped
28 ounces low-sodium, fat-free, vegetable or chicken broth
1 cup fat-free milk
1/4 teaspoon salt (optional)
1/4 teaspoon freshly ground black pepper
1/4 cup fresh chopped basil leaves
2 tablespoons chopped fresh chives

Preparation:
1. Coarsely chop tomatoes and bell peppers. Place them in a medium bowl with the corn.

2. Heat the oil in a large soup pot over medium heat. Add the onion and cook about 7 minutes or until tender, stirring occasionally.

3. Stir in tomato, pepper, scallion and corn. Cook 3 additional minutes, stirring occasionally.

4. Increase the heat to high and stir in the broth and milk. Bring to a boil. Reduce heat and simmer about 15-20 minutes or until vegetables are tender. Remove from the heat and cool for 20 minutes.

5. Once cooled, place 1/2 of vegetable mixture in a blender and process until smooth. Add the puree back to the pot. Stir in salt, black pepper, basil and chives.

DIPS

Below is a basic recipe for a dip for vegetables, bagels chips or even transformed into a salad dressing if you add a splash of vinegar, and (optional) some lite mayonnaise. It can be thinned with water, low-fat milk or even buttermilk. Mix and match the spices according to your preferences, but be aware it is easy to overdo it. Add modest amounts of spices and taste-test often.

All-Purpose Dip

1/2 cup no- or low-fat yogurt (Greek style is great)
1/2 cup low-fat sour cream
1/4 cup lite mayonnaise (optional)
Salt or celery salt to taste
Add two or more of the following options:

Chives
Chopped fresh cilantro
Chopped green onion/scallion
Chopped parsley
Crumbled feta or blue cheese
Dash of garlic powder
Dash of onion powder
Dill
Horseradish
Lemon juice or zest
Mustard
Oregano
Parmesan cheese
Other herbs and/or spices

Preparation:
1. Mix together and refrigerate a few hours before eating. Overnight is even better!

DINNER IDEAS

Cheese Fondue with Fresh Crudités and Artisan Bread
Servings: 6 (3/4 cup cheese sauce + unlimited vegetables + 1/2 cup bread cubes per serving)

1 cup low-fat milk
1 cup lite beer
2 teaspoons dry mustard
1 tablespoon Worcestershire sauce
2 cloves garlic, peeled, minced
2 tablespoons all-purpose flour
4 cups reduced-fat shredded sharp cheddar cheese
Salt and pepper to taste
Unlimited, non-starchy vegetable pieces (such as tomatoes, asparagus, cauliflower, broccoli…) Cooked protein (such as shrimp and/or chicken)
2 cups whole grain, artisan bread, cut into 2-inch cubes

Preparation:
1. In a medium bowl, toss cheese with flour until evenly coated.

2. In a medium saucepan over low heat, mix together milk, beer, Worcestershire sauce, ground dry mustard, and garlic. Heat until almost boiling.

3. Gradually stir in cheddar cheese. Continue heating mixture until all the cheese has melted.

4. Keep warm in a fondue pot or reheat and stir as needed over medium heat on the stove. Serve with cut vegetables and bread.

Classic Turkey-Vegetable Tacos
Servings: 4 (2 taco shells + half cup turkey + unlimited vegetables + 1/4 cup each shredded cheese, sour cream, and salsa per serving)

1 pound lean ground turkey
2 tablespoons chili powder
1 tablespoon ground cumin
2 teaspoons ground garlic powder

2 teaspoons ground onion powder
1/2 cup fresh cilantro
1/2 cup scallion/green onion thinly sliced
1/2 cup prepared, no-sugar-added tomato sauce
8 hard corn taco shells
2 cups romaine lettuce, shredded
2 cup diced red bell peppers
2 cups tomato, diced
1 cup red onion, diced
1 cup reduced-fat Mexican blend cheese
1 cup fat-free sour cream
1 cup all-natural, no-sugar-added salsa

Preparation:

1. Heat a medium sized skillet over medium heat. Add ground turkey and sauté until browned and most of the pink color is gone, about 8 minutes.

2. Add chili powder, cumin, garlic powder, onion powder, and tomato sauce. Cook about four more minutes or until meat is fully cooked.

3. Add green onion and cilantro. Remove from heat and keep covered until ready to use.

4. Add 1/4 cup meat to each taco shell and build tacos with vegetables based on personal preference. Serve topped with cheese, sour cream, and salsa.

Grilled Flank Steak & Portobello Stroganoff with Sun-dried Tomatoes and Barley

Servings: 4 (1 ½ cups each, plus 1/2 cup cooked barley per serving)

2 teaspoons canola oil, divided
1 tablespoon all-purpose flour
1 pound flank steak, trimmed
4 large Portobello mushrooms, stemmed, cut in half, thinly sliced
1 cup sun-dried tomatoes
1 large yellow onion, peeled, halved, thinly sliced
1 cup green bell pepper, seeded, membrane removed, diced

1 cup red bell pepper, seeded, membrane removed, diced
2 garlic cloves, minced
1 tablespoon fresh rosemary, finely chopped
1/2 cup dry red wine
2 tablespoons red wine vinegar
14 ounces of low-sodium beef broth or chicken broth
1/2 cup fat-free sour cream
1/4 cup fresh herbs such as chives, scallions, or parsley
2 cups barley, cooked

Preparation:
1. Heat outdoor grill or stovetop grill pan to medium high heat. Season steak with salt and pepper, and place it on a grill oiled with 1 teaspoon oil. Cook about 4-5 minutes on each side. Remove from heat and allow to cool. Cut into 1" pieces. Set aside until needed.

2. Heat the remaining oil in a large skillet over medium heat. Add mushrooms, onions, peppers, sun-dried tomatoes and garlic and cook stirring often until vegetables are tender and lightly browned, about 8-10 minutes. Stir in rosemary.

3. Add flour to vegetables and stir to coat. Add steak and any juices, stock, wine and vinegar and bring to a boil. Reduce heat to a simmer and cook, stirring often until mixture thickens, about 3 minutes.

4. Fold in sour cream and fresh herbs. Serve over barley.

Baked Mac & Cheese
Servings: 4

3 tablespoons plain dry breadcrumbs
1 teaspoon extra-virgin olive oil
1/4 teaspoon paprika
1 x 16-ounce or 10 ounce package frozen spinach, thawed
1 ¾ cups low-fat milk, divided
3 tablespoons all-purpose flour
2 cups shredded extra-sharp Cheddar cheese
1 cup low-fat cottage cheese

1/8 teaspoon ground nutmeg
1/4 teaspoon salt
Freshly ground pepper, to taste
8 ounces (2 cups) Dreamfields brand penne or other shape pasta

Preparation:

1. Preheat oven to 450F and bring a large pot of water to a boil. Coat an 8"-square (2-quart) baking dish with cooking spray.

2. Mix breadcrumbs, oil and paprika in a small bowl. Place spinach in a fine-mesh strainer and press out excess moisture.

3. Heat the 1 ½ cups milk in a large heavy saucepan over medium-high heat until steaming. Whisk remaining 1/4 cup milk and flour in a small bowl until smooth. Add to the hot milk and cook, whisking constantly until the sauce simmers and thickens, 2-3 minutes. Remove from heat and stir in Cheddar until melted, cottage cheese, nutmeg, salt and pepper.

4. Cook pasta for 4 minutes, or until not quite tender (it will continue to cook during baking). Drain and add to the cheese sauce, mixing well.

5. Spread half the pasta mixture in the prepared baking dish and spoon the spinach on top.

6. Top with the remaining pasta and sprinkle with the breadcrumb mixture.

7. Bake the casserole until bubbly and golden, 25-30 minutes.

White Chicken (or Turkey) Chili
Servings: 11 (one cup each)

1 tablespoon olive oil
1 ½ cups chopped onion
1/2 cup chopped celery
1/2 cup chopped red bell pepper
1 tablespoon minced seeded jalapeño pepper
1 garlic clove, minced

3 cups (about 15 ounces) chopped cooked chicken or turkey (rotisserie or precooked is fine)
2 (19-ounce) cans cannellini beans or other white beans, drained and divided
2 (16-ounce) cans fat-free, less-sodium chicken broth
1 (4.5-ounce) can chopped green chili peppers
1 cup chopped tomatoes
1 ½ teaspoons ground cumin
1 teaspoon chili powder
1 cup 1% low-fat milk
Salt and pepper to taste
1/2 cup chopped fresh cilantro
3/4 cup reduced fat white cheddar cheese (optional)

Preparation:

1. Heat olive oil in a large Dutch oven over medium-high heat. Add the onion and the

2. next 4 ingredients (celery, bell pepper, jalapeno and garlic). Sauté 5 minutes.

3. Add the chicken or turkey, 1 ½ cups beans (that's half of them), broth, and next 7 ingredients (broth, green chili peppers, tomatoes, cumin, chili pepper, salt and black pepper), and bring to a boil.

4. Cover, reduce heat and simmer 15 minutes.

5. Mash remaining beans and add them and the milk to the chicken mixture.

6. Simmer, uncovered, stirring frequently for 20 minutes or until mixture is thick.

7. Stir in chopped cilantro just before serving.

8. Top individual servings with a sprinkling of the cheddar if desired.

DESSERTS

Even children and those of us with a "sweet tooth" wouldn't complain about being served the following:

Pumpkin Pie Parfait
Servings: 10

2 x 1-ounce packages sugar-free/fat-free vanilla instant pudding
3 cups fat-free evaporated milk, chilled
1 x 15-ounce can unsweetened pumpkin
1/2 cup fat-free ricotta cheese
2 teaspoons pumpkin pie spice
1/4 cup chopped pecans, toasted
6 graham cracker squares
2 ½ cup sugar-free/fat-free whipped topping

Preparation:
1. In a medium bowl, whisk evaporated milk into vanilla instant pudding until thickened, about 4 minutes.

2. Add pumpkin, ricotta cheese and pumpkin pie spice and mix until well combined.

3. Cover and place in the refrigerator until needed.

4. In a food processor, pulse the graham crackers and toasted pecans until a crumb texture.

5. Spoon pumpkin mixture evenly among 10 serving cups. Top with 1 tablespoon crumb mixture and 1/4 cup whipped topping.

Strawberries-n-Cream
Servings: 14

1/3 cup boiling water
1 X .3-ounce package strawberry flavored sugar-free gelatin
1 X 12-ounce can fat-free evaporated milk
1/2 cup fat-free ricotta cheese
2 squares Baker's brand white chocolate
1 cup sliced strawberries

Preparation:
1. Add boiling water to gelatin and mix in medium bowl. Stir continuously for 2 minutes until completely dissolved.

2. Microwave evaporated milk and chocolate in microwaveable bowl on high for 2 minutes or until the chocolate is completely melted and mixture is well blended. Stir a few times during the 2 minutes. Add the milk mixture to the gelatin and beat with mixer until well blended.

3. Refrigerate gelatin mixture in a 9x5 inch loaf pan for 20 minutes or until firm.

4. Unmold gelatin mixture when solid and cut into 14 rectangles.

5. Top each rectangle with sliced strawberries.

Lemon Chiffon with Red Grapes and Walnuts
Servings: 10

1/2 cup boiling water
1 x .3-ounce package sugar-free lemon flavored gelatin
1/2 cup seedless red grapes, halved
1/4 cup fat-free sour cream
3 tablespoons chopped walnuts, toasted

Preparation:
1. Add boiling water to the gelatin mix and stir 2 minutes until completely dissolved.

2. Allow to stand at room temperature until almost cool.

3. Whisk sour cream into cooled gelatin in a bowl until well blended. Pour into a 9-inch square pan and top with grapes and walnuts.

4. Refrigerate about 1 hour or until firm.

Chocolate-Peanut Butter Mousse
Servings: 10

2 x 1.4-ounce packages sugar-free/fat-free instant chocolate pudding
2 cups fat-free milk

1/2 cup all-natural, creamy peanut butter
1 ½ cups lite whipped topping, thawed
1/4 cup semi-sweet chocolate chips
1/4 cup chopped roasted, unsalted peanuts

Preparation:
1. Whisk pudding mix, milk and peanut butter in a medium bowl until well combined and thickened, about 4 minutes.

2. Stir in whipped topping.

3. Pour into a 9-inch square pan. Top with semi-sweet chocolate chips and chopped roasted unsalted peanuts.

4. Refrigerate for 1 hour before serving.

Red, White, and Blueberry Panna Cotta
Servings: 6

1 cup + 3 tablespoons skim milk
1 envelope unflavored gelatin
1/4 cup maple syrup, or honey, or Splenda brand sweetener
1 teaspoon vanilla extract
2 cups fat-free plain Greek yogurt
1 ½ cups strawberries, hulled, quartered
1 ½ cups fresh blueberries

Preparation
1. In a small bowl, sprinkle the gelatin over the 3 tablespoons of milk and allow to rest and soften for about 5 minutes.

2. Meanwhile, in a saucepan, heat the remaining 1 cup of milk until it is simmering, but do not let it boil. Add the vanilla and honey and stir to combine.

3. Whisk in the gelatin and continue to whisk until it has completely melted into the hot milk.

4. Stir in the yogurt and mix until well combined.

5. Pour 1/2 cup of the mixture into each of the 6 x 1 cup glasses. Refrigerate for at least 3-4 hours.

6. Top each cup with the strawberries and blueberries.

You can plan your meals ahead of time, shop and stock your shelves accordingly, but there is no way to avoid being surrounded by food. Great efforts are made to entice us to eat. Even in our own homes we are bombarded by commercials on TV, watch actors dine, and hear food references constantly. Further, the minute we leave our homes we are bombard by even more stimuli that encourages us to eat. Ads, aromas, and even socializing often involve food. Food is everywhere in our environment, so we'll want to put some thought into how we deal with this onslaught!

☆   ☆   ☆

Chapter 8

TAKE CHARGE OF YOUR FOOD ENVIRONMENT

We are surrounded by food, people, and events that bring food and people together. Like a clock, food related activities designate the time of day, such as dinner *time*, rest *time*, lunch *hour*, nap *time*, play *time*, relaxation *time*, etc. Because of this, food controls and measures the flow and pace of our lives; it anchors us. Some of us even dream of food. Time is often described as a flowing river. More than a few of us view time as a smorgasbord on a conveyer belt. If we're trying to control our diabetes and lose weight, this is a problem. To be successful, we'll want to take charge of our food environment.

Mealtimes, for some of us, are the most important events of the day, and we often start thinking about our next meal before we polish off the one in front of us. The proverbial deck seems to be stacked against us, so we have to use every trick in the book from profound to simple to deal with this tempting conveyor belt and the brilliant minds of a well equipped army of marketing professionals who stop at nothing to get us to buy and eat their foods. We can win this battle if we outsmart them, but we'll have to be very cunning and stick to our guns.

We can talk about our food environment and we can talk about our social environment, but it is sometimes impossible to separate the two. Food brings people together as well as expresses our feelings for people. Food, more often than not, is something to be shared. It is downright rude, for example, to eat in front of others without at least offering to share what we have, even if our offer is obviously insincere. Who is really going to say "yes" to an offer to nibble the south end of your sardine sandwich? Food has such a strong social association, some people refuse to eat alone in a restaurant unless it is a fast food joint. They fear it appears they have no one with whom to dine. Eating, like religion, also has its own rituals, from who carves the turkey to the proper placement of eating utensils. Its similarity to religion doesn't end here. More than a couple of us have fallen on our knees in rapture when an extra large slice of chocolate layer cake appears. We even say it tastes, "Heavenly"! Chocolates, of course, say, "I love you," and cakes say, "Congratulations"! Sayings such as, "A way to a man's heart is through his stomach," are powerful, if not true. To reject an offering of food is usually perceived as a personal insult, and to not offer food is a way of telling someone they are intruding.

Let's break this confusing food-social environment down into smaller portions and come up with suggestions on how to handle some of the real situations we face. We'll look at everything from meal planning and buying food to tricks for family dining. Don't worry if you live alone, there are some tips for you here too. Because others around us inevitably respond to our change in diet and lifestyle, we'll explore common reactions, from those who support our efforts to change, to those who sabotage our every step. Also, many of us want a few tricks that get us through special events such as social gatherings and vacations. We want to be prepared to handle them all, because we'll probably encounter them all. Most of all, we want to be able to fully enjoy life's wonderful social events and people without being undermined by our new lifestyle. We can do both. After all, if our new lifestyle isn't a trade up, isn't a better life, then what's the point?

SHOPPING AND FOOD SELECTION

We all know not to shop when we're hungry. We've all learned that the hard way, even though we often ignore our own guidance. Sometimes, due to other demands on our time, we have little control over when we shop. However, the more control we have over the food that enters our home, the better off we are. If you don't do the food shopping, it might be high time to volunteer for the job. If you do all the shopping for the family, you already have control over much of what comes into your home, and you're off to a good start.

Where you live affects your accessibility to healthy foods, especially fresh produce. There are inner city areas where fresh vegetables are hard to find, and when they are found, they are often overpriced and are of inferior quality. This lack of availability creates a significant burden for many, and is especially hard for those of us trying to lose weight and control our diabetes. Further, in some locales, it is cheaper to feed a family from a chain's calorie packed "dollar menu" than purchase fresh meat and vegetables locally. However, there are many inspiring accounts of inner city neighbors joining forces to purchase vegetables in large quantities from outside their immediate neighborhood by setting up food cooperatives. If you live in an area that lacks fresh food, check around to see if there is an active cooperative you can join. If there isn't one, consider starting one. Yes, seriously! Alternatively, you may have to devote more time to shopping because of the need to travel some distance to find the foods you want. Planning ahead is therefore all the more important. The lack of availability of some foods also holds true for those of us living in rural areas; the local store might be many miles away and the availability of fresh produce and meats might be extremely limited. In contrast, there are areas where fresh vegetables grow all year long, and the availability and price inspires creative cooking. This has led to the development of new cuisines, such as "Southern California Cuisine," for example. Bottom line is that some of us have to work harder to get healthy food into our homes than others. Do whatever you must to get the food you require to make your weight loss and diabetes control efforts pay off.

SML MEALS ARE GOOD FOR THE WHOLE FAMILY

Although we're attempting to take more control over our environment, remember a diet based on balancing SML carbs is a good diet for the whole family, so don't you dare feel guilty for introducing this way of eating to your household! You are doing something good for all members, so consider presenting it that way! If you start off by preparing (or having someone prepare) some of the more popular meals without guilt or apologies, family members will be more likely to not only support but also encourage your efforts to change your lifestyle. Planning your meals and snacks in advance, and shopping only for the ingredients in those meals, gives you great control over what enters your home. Food, in spite of some spurious allegations, does not walk into your home on its own. However, we can all attest that it does disappear "into thin air" on occasion. Take as much control over the food entering your home as you can, and you'll be helping yourself and all others in your household. In fact, consider making meal planning, shopping and cooking a family event. Almost everyone can benefit from learning these skills; they can take their lessons with them through life.

SHORT-ACTING FOOD AND SHORT-TERM THINKING: A DIABOLICAL DUO

Short-acting foods (simple carbs) are foods we crave to satisfy our hunger when we can't think beyond our immediate urge to satisfy our intense cravings. When we are ravenous, our brain could care less about our long-term plans and commitments. One important thing to keep in mind is that we sometimes eat simply because the food is there. The mere presence of food is a cue to eat; it beckons us, and some of us swear we can hear it call our name from another room. Remember, in the presence of food, our ancient ancestor feast or famine programmed brain says, "Hey, you better chow down; there's probably a famine around the corner!" Of course, we're all more than happy to comply. You have some options for how you control foods that seem to entice your short-term thinking from entering your home:

Snack Outings

One successful approach is to ask family members or those with whom you reside to go out for the foods and snacks they enjoy but you do not want them around. If food is not available, you won't eat it. If family members want special snacks, have them go out for them and eat them before they come home. The last thing you want is a large, industrial size box of your favorite cookies on a shelf whispering your name day and night. It may cost more per cookie for a household member to buy small portions to eat out-side the home, but if doing so helps you get healthier, it is a bargain. Remember, if "decadent" food items are not available, you will not eat them.

Food Security Pat Downs

If you can't get family members to go out for their special treats, you might be tempted to take control over food entering your home by instituting a "pat down" procedure for all those who enter. Of course, you'll have to endure being called "warden" (or worse), especially if you insist on wearing a Taser gun on your belt as a fashion accessory. Unfortunately, strangers entering your home might misunderstand your physical pat downs, or worse, start dropping by more frequently once word gets out! Finally, there is nothing worse than ill-timed photos of your meticulous frisks appearing on Facebook! Perhaps a more moderate approach is better.

The Conspiratorial Approach to Food Control

Having all but ruled out the option of pat downs (please agree you have), there must be a better way to prevent certain foods from entering your home. You can issue an edict, and make a list of the "forbidden" foods, but we all know household members will attempt to cheat. If you are adamant enough, your diligence will insure they become expert at sneaking food in. You can be assured they'll hide it outside your sight and grasp. This approach will work for you, because food items will be unavailable to you. But this approach only works if your family members are especially gifted in the refined art of deceit and deception, not the best character traits for you to encourage unless you're in the "grifter" trade and consider such lessons homeschooling. Worse, this approach falls apart when you see them wearing winter coats in the middle of summer just to smuggle in food. A cake box under a parka fools no one. Bottom line is that requiring family members to be deceitful is wrong, especially if they are children. There must be a better way.

The Cooperative and Supportive Approach

If you approach the basic "concept" of deterring "elicit" foods from entering your home, but do so in an open and honest manner, you can still get the more mature family members to agree to hide their special stash from you. Just let them know you want their help to avoid temptation, and that the availability of food is a strong temptation. Honesty is the best policy. Yes, you will have to ask them to hide their stash in areas you would not stumble upon accidently and agree is off limits. You must also agree, in turn, to respect their privacy and not adopt a bloodhound to aid you in finding their hidden stash. If you start snooping, you'll blow it, you'll breach the agreement. If they are children and are too young to participate in your scheme, simply take them out for special treats. You'll be more successful at tolerating short intervals of temptation than trying to relax while delectable edibles entice you from within walking distance. Actually, you might want to join the kids in a treat once in a while when out. Just be reasonable and have one scoop of no sugar added ice cream instead of trying to create a totem pole on a cone. Always remember, you want a lifestyle that allows you to enjoy life. Consistency is more important than perfection. Eventually, you'll make the transition in your head from "diet" to "lifestyle". It takes time and practice, but it comes with time.

No Guilt Allowed

Again, because it bears repeating, don't feel guilty about taking control over the food in your home or improving your life. Your actions are not selfish. Don't underestimate the importance of a good diet in everyone's life. Family members can always opt for larger portions and personalize their diet, but it is not like you are expecting them to partake in some bizarre or unorthodox food fetish. In fact, you might be helping other household members establish healthier eating habits, not to mention the importance of serving as a good role model for personal achievement— something never to be underestimated.

LIVING ALONE

Living alone sounds ideal when it comes to controlling the food that enters your home, but those of us living alone face different problems. We too know that if food is available, we'll eat it, and many foods are not portioned for individual servings. It is common practice to eat double or more portions because of the size container in which food is available. Because of this, it is easy for us to eat more, sometimes simply because we want to eat our food before it spoils. It is forbidden in most if not all cultures to waste food (unless it is sacrificed). Strangely, we will often knowingly allow food products to turn unnatural colors before we are willing to throw them away. We seem to provide a special "wake period" for food—a period of time between when you refuse to eat something because it is too old to safely consume, and the time you feel you *must* discard it. Food wakes usually go on for days, sometimes longer. If you live alone, you have to get over this. You are probably going to have to throw out more food, so change your mind-set. Do not consider it "wasting," consider it "recycling". Eating food to avoid throwing it out is not going to feed a single child in any third world country, regardless of what your momma told you. In addition, you can decrease the amount of discarded food if you find someone with whom to share food. In some cases, shopping more frequently helps you conserve food. For example, buying single serving sizes of vegetables rather than price-conscious larger bags helps prevent having to discard food. Although the extra cost of buying some food from the salad bar seems a waste of money, if you end up eating it all and not throwing some out, it might actually save you money. If it doesn't end up saving you money, consider it money well spent anyway. Do not let living alone provide you with a built in excuse. You have many things working in your favor, so take full advantage of them.

FAMILIES

Each family is different. Some are fortunate enough to be able to gather at designated times such as evening meals. This works out well, because there are some wonderful SML dishes that will satisfy any family. You can build around the SML meals to allow individuals to cater to their special likes and dislikes. One of the keys to success is to take the extra time required to prepare meals that the whole family will enjoy. This is especially true in the beginning when family members' resistance is at its highest. Preparing double portions and freezing one also helps.

To make your SML meal work for all, you'll want to plan in advance, and in some cases, drop some of the spontaneity of meal preparation you've practiced in the past. "Spontaneity" too often results in calling out for a pizza or Chinese food, and such occasions are treated like both time-savers and indulgent celebrations. Every family benefits from having a few backup "quick meals" that fit into the SML approach. Get used to "throwing them together," instead of dialing. Just getting the food strategy figured out is hard enough, but some families also have some "non-edible" problems that interfere with our efforts to lose weight.

FAMILY AND FRIEND'S REACTIONS TO YOUR NEW LIFESTYLE

Inevitably, family, friends, and maybe coworkers, will react to your efforts to lose weight and create a new lifestyle. This is especially true if you share social activities with them that involve food. Before we look at how people may react to your change in diet, don't forget that they too may be influenced by some of the common negative stereotypes of heavy people that exist. Their stereotypes may not only influence how they view you, but also how they view themselves. Keep in mind that, although common, not everyone has negative stereotypes or prejudices against heavy people; in fact there are signs that things are changing. The most common negative stereotype is that people who are overweight lack control. Another variation of this theme is that fat people are lazy and sloppy. Some people even think that large people, especially women, are not as smart as thin women. Unfortunately, many of us heavy people also believe these negative stereotypes about ourselves, especially if we believe our weight is a result of the lack of willpower! But hey, we don't need others to humiliate us if we're doing a fine job ourselves! It is important for everyone, including ourselves, to know these negative stereotypes are simply not true!

In general, women tend to be weight conscious whereas men are more physique conscious. You only have to look to male sports figures to see why physique rather than weight is the standard of measurement. There are other differences between men and women. For example, it is much harder for fat women to hold positions of power than it is for fat men. Look at members of congress for example, or think of the stereotypical banker. There are always exceptional people who break through the negative stereotypes, but if you start to name them you'll discover a short list. Go ahead, Oprah...

Thin women, on the other hand are seen as powerful and in control. The peer pressure to be thin, especially in some social and professional circles, is severe. The country club crowd is a good example of this. Although there are some naturally thin people, there are also those whose thinness is the result of constant vigilance and extreme denial of their hunger. They obsess over their food intake and their exercise. Sadly, many thin women are not really "allowed" to fess up to their peers about how difficult it is to remain thin. Admitting it is hard work is usually socially unacceptable—a confession of weakness. They'll nibble on a salad and proclaim to their friends that they are "naturally light eaters". Sometimes they even convince themselves they are. They are not without their negative stereotype either. Describing someone as "skinny" often is followed by "bitch". In fact, their disposition might indeed be influenced by chronic low blood sugar due to their extreme diet and exercise. Unfortunately, their great success at weight maintenance is often offset by the lack of happiness in their lives. It is simply not a good way to live. At times, their obsession can even turn into a serious eating disorder.

Your family, friends and coworkers might be influenced by negative stereotypes as much as the next person, even though they love you. Because every person is unique, so too will be his or her reaction to your change in diet and lifestyle.

Typical Reactions

Some people will support your efforts and some not. Some reactions (or lack of a reaction) might best be ignored, while others might best be confronted. Most reactions, you'll realize, fall into one of five categories below…more or less. Here are some common reactions as well as a few tips on how to handle people who seem to fit into each of the following five categories:

1. The Aiders and Abettors

Many people have issues with food and a number of them will feel you are abandoning them for your new lifestyle. Remember that food and social activities are interlinked, and if you change one, you might also end up changing the other. There is sometimes a secret fear that your new lifestyle will negatively affect your relationship. You know that many reactions come from the family and friends' insecurities, and that's important to keep in mind. Aiders and abettors are usually not mean spirited, and they often express (in words or actions) their philosophy: "You should love your large body and enjoy life and food." They interpret your desire to change as coming from self-rejection rather than an acceptance of your potential. This helps them justify not dealing with their own problems…but that's okay. They don't want to see you struggle, but more important, they also don't want to look like a failure in comparison to your accomplishments. Some will actually say, "Good luck but don't expect me to go along with this." It becomes obvious that many of them are struggling with their own weight issue. If they are skilled, they'll pluck your strings just the right way and persuade you to eat decadent foods with them. They like to entice you to "cheat" (as they see it), and make the indulgence sound very attractive, a valued treat, playful, and even naughty. Some will say, "Let yourself go, be free, enjoy, and love yourself for who you are!"

Because they know how to get to you, and eventually probably will wear you down if you don't take action, you'll have to address the problem. Of course, this assumes you want to retain your relationship with them. You must talk to them. Make your "chat" clear, simple, and unapologetic. Most important, do not criticize them, even if you want to smack them one. Here's a quick guideline for your "little talk":

A. Let them know how much you value or love them and how important they are to you. Do not lay it on too thick; keep it real.
B. Let them know you are putting a great deal of effort into creating a new lifestyle, and your commitment is coming out of self-respect and self-love.
C. Let them know that regardless of the well-intentioned "invitations," they work against your effort, and you find them uncomfortable.
D. Let them know you would greatly appreciate their support.
E. Be specific about how they can help. Give them directions and examples. Many people don't know how to give support without specific requests—it is simply too general a request. Focus on what they can do to help you rather than what they "should" or "shouldn't" do.
F. Get them to verbally agree. Ask, "So, are you willing to help me this way?" If they hesitate or change the subject, it means "no". Let it go.
G. If they agree but later screw up, remind them, forgive them, but keep an eye on them.

Of course, you'll handle it like a pro and they'll grow to not only admire you, but they might also follow in your path one day on their own mission to improve their life. Recruit them by example, not harassment or embarrassment. Of course, some who fit this category simply don't give much thought to their reaction to you. Some individuals, however, can be downright harmful.

2. Undermining Family and Friends

It is sad that we have to cover this, but there are people who might undermine your lifestyle change efforts. They are like the above group, but more harmful, they are extreme examples of the above. More often than not, they have their own personal issues, but it can get pretty intense if you are close to them.

Your diabetes control and weight loss are health issues. No one is allowed to sabotage your health…no one. You can't allow anyone to encourage you to cause physical damage to yourself. Regardless of their own personal issues, and your sensitivity and understanding toward them, you have to either stop them or totally ignore them—if that is possible. If talking to them following the above guidelines doesn't work, and it is possible it won't work, say goodbye to them. In some cases they'll be shocked into "seeing the light" and in other cases they will not. So be it.

It is much harder if the undermining person is a family member. Although some people have no qualms about cutting off family members, most of us try to maintain "good enough" relationships within the family for the sake of other family members. If the person undermining you is a member of your immediate household, you must certainly be aware of the effects upon you of living in such a tense or even noxious environment. It is simply not good for your health. Sometimes, however, we have limited options, but many times we are unable to even recognize our options. We might benefit from help to find our way out of the mess. Reality really sucks at times.

Other than severing relationships, there are no quick, one-shot remedies to this serious problem. Realize first that more often than not, their reaction is about you changing and growing without them. They may fear being left behind, or worse, they may feel they're losing you. Let them know you won't let them undermine your efforts (use polite words and wait until you feel relatively calm and not angry to have your chat). Hold your ground. On occasion, time itself helps people see things more clearly. If you can, maintain your composure and do not retaliate with negativity. Don't let them sway you away from your commitment. They might…just might…be encouraged to deal with their own issue or at least back off…kind of an unspoken truce. Occasionally, over time, they might come to realize their fear is irrational. By holding your ground and not overreacting, they may slowly become more aware of their own behavior.

In some cases, even parents will undermine their adult (and sometimes very mature) children's efforts to improve their lives. This can happen at any age, and it is very painful. Some parents see their children's attempts to change as a rejection of them and their parenting skills. For example, they may feel guilty that the way they raised you might be responsible for your excess weight, or fear you secretly hold them responsible. Show compassion and understanding toward them, but once again, dig in your heels. Don't be surprised if they go underground and play on your vulnerabilities, including guilt, or instigate sibling rivalry. Remind yourself that they aren't bad parents if they raised you to be strong enough to change your life. Do not retaliate by withholding love or gifts. They really could use those new slippers you were going to buy.

3.   The Indifferent Friend or Family Member

Well, at least the indifferent ones are not undermining you! Indifference can feel surprisingly hurtful, at times worse than even anger. It is the apparent lack of interest in you and the failure to connect or care about you that hurts deeply. Some people simply don't appreciate our efforts, but that does not make them bad people. They might not be able to relate to your struggle, or simply lack the ability to be empathetic. Their reaction may have less to do with you than you think. Many people are so into their own worlds, our world is unimportant and invisible to them. Alternately, they may just be playing it safe and don't want to have to deal with either your successes or failures; they just want to stay neutral and safe. There is a difference between disinterest and neutrality. In any case, you'll find others who support and appreciate you. Just don't let their indifference or neutrality change the way you view yourself or your commitment to improve your life.

4. The Annoying Encouragers

The big problem with annoying encouragers is that they make it harder for us to fail. How dare they! Their heads and hearts are probably in a very good place, and we want to appreciate them for that. They can become our mainstay and remind us of our long-term goals when we're tempted to only think about the immediate future. Some of us less secure folks may feel a bit annoyed by their over enthusiasm, because we perceive it as a rejection of the way we currently are or were. We sort of hear, "Oh, thank heaven you're finally changing!" Yes, it is double sided, and yes you'll imagine hearing their nagging voice whenever a dessert tray passes you, but take the encouragers for who they are and their importance in your life. Once they see you don't want constant encouragement (or nagging or guilt trips), they might settle down. Certainly, you can find the right moment and words to ask them to "lighten up" a bit. Tapering your responses to their encouragements, or ignoring them altogether also discourages them. Just don't be rude about it and risk losing their support. In the long run, they will probably feel part of your success and it would be gracious of you to one day credit some of your success to their support. Maybe, just maybe, they believe in you and want to share in your success. There's nothing wrong with that.

5. Non-Judgmental Lifestyle Change Supporters

Keep them near and dear. Collect more of them. Return their support twofold, and put them in your will.

SPOUSES AND PARTNERS

You really want your spouse or partner on your side. It is best if they are totally involved. If you are out to lose weight and they are not, make it a joint "healthy lifestyle change," or "life-satisfaction boost". Don't limit it to a "diabetes control and weight loss" project.

For insecure spouses, the idea of their partner changing in any way can be very threatening. They have a choice of letting it motivate them or scare them. It is not uncommon for spouses or partners to somehow fear your efforts will be so successful that you will "trade them in" for a better model. You might want to allow things a little time to "settle down" and let them realize that your venture is not the threat they imagine. Insecurities aside, if your partner or spouse doesn't support your efforts to improve your health, you have a problem in your relationship more serious than their reaction to your new venture. It is just a symptom of a larger problem, and it may be time to consult a professional.

HANDLING SPECIAL GATHERINGS AND OCCASIONS

Family gatherings and celebrations of all sorts bring out the tastiest foods, and they often take center stage. It is sometimes suggested that you try to time your arrival to either before or after the food is served, but that is usually difficult and it takes away much of the joy. Arriving at unusual times can also annoy people or be misinterpreted. It is better to remind yourself that you can join the gathering and enjoy the festivities as well as food without bingeing. Just use some common sense restraint and use your food diary. Your food diary will serve you much better than abandoning your new lifestyle for the day. Snacking on medium-acting carbs a couple hours before you leave for the event can help, but remember that you are trying to build a lifestyle full of joy. Denying yourself satisfaction at special events is not helping you develop a durable lifestyle. In many cases, you can scan your food options and put together a respectable enough SML meal. It might not be perfect, but you're not aiming for perfection. Remember, enjoying life and being happy is good for your weight loss and diabetes control!

You can increase your enjoyment by focusing on the pleasure you get from being around friends and relatives rather than thinking constantly about the food that's available. Often, food takes center stage and without it, no one would show up at some social events! Don't fall into the trap of viewing gatherings as an excuse to overeat. Also, don't forget your biology wants you to eat simply because food is present. During your extended social festivities, you might run into your cousin Agnes who eats like a horse and gains nothing!

There is no value in comparing yourself with her or anyone else like her, for that matter. There are people who have freaky metabolisms, and that's just the way it goes. However, do not call Agnes a "freak of nature" at family events or try to force-feed her out of revenge. It's just not right.

AROMA AVOIDANCE

Be careful about entering bakeries without an armed guard…to protect others from you! Smell is an overwhelmingly powerful sense that is hotwired to primitive parts of our brains. You can probably detect cinnamon wafting through the air by just reading about it. You may also be salivating on this page. Sorry.

DINING OUT

Restaurants have gotten savvier over the years and know they have to cater to dieters of all types. More often than not, they offer an adequate selection of healthy foods. If not, suggest a different restaurant. There is no reason you can't stick to your SML meal plan when eating out. Sure you might have to decide between either the bread or the potato, and you might have to ask to substitute one of them for a side of vegetables, but it can usually be done and you can still enjoy your meal. You may also decide to share a main entre and double up on a side order, or turn an appetizer into a main dish. Don't be timid about making special requests. If you don't get wait staff to run back to the kitchen to, "ask the chef" a couple of times, you really must sharpen up your act! Denying yourself the enjoyment of dining out isn't a good idea; it is actually a bad one. Food isn't the only source of pleasure when you eat out. The dining atmosphere, being served, no dishes to clean, and great company all bring much, if not more pleasure than the food itself! You want your new lifestyle to add satisfaction to your life, not diminish it. This doesn't mean you want to throw caution to the wind and abandon your diet either. A common sense approach to dining out is the way to go and fits nicely into your new lifestyle. As for your food diary, you know the answer!

VACATIONS, OUTINGS AND EXCURSIONS

Be it a vacation, or just a day in the countryside (or city) the whole purpose of an escape is often just to get away from the demands and routines of daily life. It is extremely tempting to "give yourself a break," from your food diary too, but doing so can lead to habits that sabotage your long-term goal. Think of vacations and excursions as extended dining out experiences! Do not take a vacation from your SML meal plans, because you do not take a vacation from a lifestyle. Use a common sense approach, but add a little more planning to it. When possible, decide what you're eating plans are for the day, so you won't be caught off guard, and so you can "pace" and better plan your meals. The one thing you may be tempted to do, but absolutely don't want to do, is take a vacation from your food diary. It is far better to keep track of a not-so-proud eating day than not keep track of it. Actually, you'll find the "binge" diaries help you change more than the "kale and sprouts" diary.

Vacations are actually a time to celebrate your weight loss. Be aware of how many more activities you can enjoy, how much better you move, and how much more comfortable and attractive you are becoming. Those are the real rewards, the real payoffs, and they will influence your meal choices more than anything! Rather than seeing vacations as threats to your new way of eating, see them as your reward, your opportunity to see and feel the benefits of your new lifestyle. Keeping it positive makes it all much easier.

It is wonderful to celebrate weight loss, and most of us are going to slim down simply by sticking to the SML meal plans. A few of us, however, may find we are not losing weight or not losing weight fast enough. There are a few different way to increase the speed of your weight loss, and it is time to share those tips with you.

✳   ✳   ✳

Chapter 9

POWERFUL TIPS TO ACCELERATE WEIGHT LOSS

Success breeds success, and if you start losing weight soon after you start on the SML (Short-Medium-Long) meal plan you'll be more strongly motivated to stick to it. Some of us may be so encouraged by our initial weight loss, we want to speed it up! On the other extreme unfortunately, some of us find that our impressive initial weight loss slows down or even appears to halt. Although we'll explore this particularly frustrating situation shortly, here are some tips to help all of us lose weight regardless of our motivation:

1. If you stick to your SML meal plan and keep your daily calorie counts below the calories you burn, you'll lose weight. It may not be dramatic, but you will slowly lose weight. An ideal pace to lose weight is about one pound a week.

2. Remember scales are dirty liars! Actually, they don't lie…it is just that we misinterpret what they are telling us. Aside from being somewhat inaccurate, and being fussy about how they are placed, all they measure is overall weight. Weight includes not only fat, but water, muscle, bones, and your organs. If you are exercising more, you might be adding weight to your muscles and therefore compensating for the loss of fat. Water plays an even bigger role, and your water content can change daily. Scales that measure not only weight, but fat and water, called "bioelectrical impedance analysis" or BIA scales, will give you a more accurate picture. Remember you want to lose fat, and fat is just one of the component of weight. Because electricity travels through water, but not fat, it is able to measure the percentage of fat in your body and the percentage of water. The scale, which also measures your overall weight, does some calculations and tells you the percentage of fat you

have. BIA scales are more accurate than traditional scales, and there are many types from which to choose, ranging in price from $30 to $400. Except for the most expensive ones, they are not accurate if you are dehydrated, and some of the inexpensive ones aren't any more accurate than regular scales.

3. Losing weight is not a smooth, steady decline. No, that would make it too easy for us! If you weigh yourself every day, you'll see this. There are ups and downs on a daily and weekly basis that don't seem to make sense. Many of these changes are very discouraging, especially if you see your weight increasing in spite of your efforts. If we let it, our mood can go up and down along with the numbers on the scale. Weighing yourself every day is almost as bad as strapping a scale to each foot and looking down at them to check your weight throughout the day. Weighing yourself less often, perhaps once each week or once each month, makes more sense. This annoying weight fluctuation has led some of us to forgo scales altogether (unless they are in a doctor's office), and judge our progress by how our clothes fit. The fancier BIA scales made for home use that measure not only overall weight, but also body fat and water, also have the same fluctuations. Some scales are so bad they ought to be sold with a free exorcism coupon!

4. We've all been on those crash diets and are accustomed to losing 2 or 3 pounds and maybe even more during the first week. This is deceiving, because body fat and weight loss don't correlate well, especially when beginning a diet. On most diets, as soon as you begin, your body uses the sugar stored in your liver and muscles. The sugar stored there is called glycogen. Each glycogen molecule is surrounded by water, which is pulled out along with the sugar. This can amount to 5 to 10 lbs of weight loss! No wonder we're sold on those diets! You will start losing real body fat only after that supply of glycogen is used up. You'll lose it steadily if you eat approximately 500 calories less than you burn each day, but how much you actually lose also depends on your metabolic rate (the rate at which you burn calories).

5. You probably only want to lose about a pound a week. That's a nice, reasonable loss, and folks who lose weight at this rate stand a better chance of keeping it off.

If you want to accelerate your diet, there are things you can do. They include:

1. Keeping a food diary
2. Keeping an exercise diary in addition to your food diary
3. Counting calories consumed
4. Determining the calories you burn each day
5. Completing an extreme hunger analysis and management plan
6. Having wine for dessert...maybe

THE POWER OF A FOOD DIARY

There are two types of people who use the SML approach to weight loss: those who keep food diaries and those who don't. Those who use food diaries see progress and can continue to lose weight on their own after an average of 12 weeks. Generally speaking, they make the successful transition in their approach to eating and diabetes management. At about three months, they have the tools they require to continue to lose weight on their own. They even send holiday cards with updates on their progress each year thanking those who helped them make this major lifestyle change. They often enclose photos showing off their new bodies. Keeping a food diary is as close to magic as it gets, but...

Who in their right mind wants to keep a food diary? There are at least ten rational reasons why this is a stupid waste of time. Common sense tells us this! On an emotional level, it feels like we're being asked to hand in a school paper for a grade, or report to a boss who doesn't even have us on their payroll! It feels belittling, manipulative and disrespectful...but, by golly, it works! People who don't keep food diaries can make progress, but it is measured across years, not months.

Whenever "diary refusers" are captured and interrogated long enough under a bare, bright light (swaying, of course, at the end of a long cord from the ceiling of a small, stuffy room), they always admit through their annoying snivels that they hate food diaries. They whine about their bad experiences with them; or worse, they think diaries are about increasing their consciousness or creating some weird form of accountability to an authority figure standing in judgment. Once their protests are aired, their written confessions signed, and their pathetic sobbing has subsided, it is time to dim the light, give them a sugar-free ice tea, and open the window to let in some fresh air.

Given a voice, the fresh air would probably say: We all want pride, but your pride is getting in the way, my friend; in this instance, you may want to think of it as possibly being false pride. What are you really protesting? It is not a belittling, futile, useless exercise unless you have firmly decided it will become so, in which case you'll get what you want. More important, you are probably reacting this way based on misinformation—very common misinformation actually, so don't feel "bad" about it. The food diary isn't about raising conscious- ness or about adding some external form of control at all; it is about engaging parts of your brain that have not been involved in food planning, food choice, or eating activities. It changes "I will eat this," into "I will eat this and I will write it down." Writing down your food intake will increase your eating expertise. Writing it down helps you store that information in more parts of the brain, and in effect, aids your thinking and helps you change your behavior. The practice is indeed brain food. As just one example (and there are many!) of how your brain is affected, remember taking notes in school? You didn't always go back to read them, did you? Fess up! When it came to a quiz, you often remembered what you wrote, not what the teacher said! The same learning takes place when using a food diary. The informa- tion you retrieved for those tests was stored in different areas of your brain than the original point the teacher made! You could probably even recall if the answer was written on the right or left page of your tattered, doodle-filled notebook, how far down the note was from the top of the page, and what color ink was used! Now that's using your head! The more you use your head, the more successful you will be at weight loss! If you were more studious, you might have actu- ally reviewed your notes, and discovered you were reminding your- self of what you remembered—committing the information into a more permanent form of memory. You would have been making new associations to that distinct piece of memory, and that would have aided your learning, retention, and recall. Learning, it seems, is quite complex, and there are even more arguments to be made—but you'll be spared. This brief lecture on how memory works aside, you must admit that those in your class who wrote and reviewed their notes did better and got better grades than those who didn't. That's all that is important. Don't even think about bringing up Johnny what's-his-name from the 7th grade who memorized a whole set of encyclopedias! That is unfair and uncalled for, and very defensive! Johnny was an exception, a genius, and one in a million! That little twerp probably owns half of Florida by now!

You are not entering a contest or competing against anyone with your diary entries. If by keeping a diary you are afraid you will not live up to your own expectations, give yourself a break. It is not about shaming yourself into changing your diet. Sometimes we're so afraid of failure that it is safer not to try. It is easier to call yourself "stubborn" or "lazy" than a "failure"—it has less of a sting—so, please don't think of the food diary in a negative way. Actually, when keeping your food diary, the most important days are those days when you don't meet your goals! How are you to learn if not by your mistakes? You are not only allowed to make mistakes, they are required! You will learn a little each time you make one. Even when your food diary entries become somewhat predictable, or even if you are pleased with your food intake and you are on a roll, keep your food diary going; it is the consistency and the willingness to make it a daily practice that supports your commitment and helps you change your life. It is a wonderful tool that works on many levels, and the importance of keeping a food diary can't be overstated. It becomes easier over time, and is really not very hard. Considering the alternatives, it is "a piece of cake"!

Your Diary Format

The format of your diary matters. Generally, the simpler the diary, the better. Don't get too caught up using the most advanced technology, unless you find it motivating (which many people do). You want something simple, user friendly, and most important, accessible. If you use a computer to access your diary and you are not in front of one much of the day, it probably isn't the best way to keep a diary. Having to sign on to a site on the Internet in order to enter your food intake may be just that extra step or two that results in your efforts falling apart. Having 100% access to your food diary, with the minimal amount of effort, is the key to success. Your choice depends on your lifestyle. Here are some options:

Paper and Pen

This is the most common sense method, because it is readily available; easily transportable, inexpensive, doesn't use electricity, is biodegradable, and doesn't require frequent upgrades or antivirus programs. Simply jot down the time, what you ate, and if you choose, the approximate amount of calories. Adding up the calories for the day is helpful for many. Start the next day with a new date right under yesterday's diary entries.

For example:

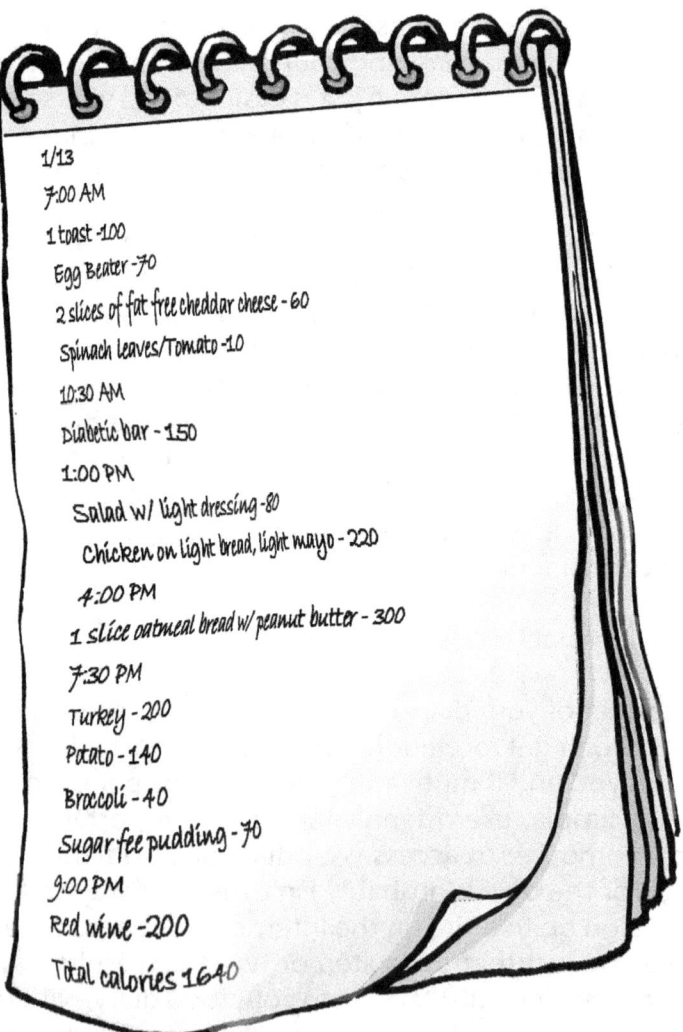

1/13
7:00 AM
1 toast -100
Egg Beater -70
2 slices of fat free cheddar cheese - 60
Spinach leaves/Tomato -10
10:30 AM
Diabetic bar - 150
1:00 PM
Salad w/ light dressing -80
Chicken on light bread, light mayo - 220
4:00 PM
1 slice oatmeal bread w/ peanut butter - 300
7:30 PM
Turkey - 200
Potato - 140
Broccoli - 40
Sugar free pudding - 70
9:00 PM
Red wine -200
Total calories 1640

Common Computer Software and Independent of the Internet

There are many software programs such as word processing programs that can be used for your diary. You can use "insert table" to create a nice grid. Some folks prefer to keep their food diary in the "notes" function of software schedulers, many of which sync with wireless devices. They do everything but prepare your meal and wash the dishes. Some tech savvy people simply use a standard database. Even for them, keeping it easy and accessible is the key.

Internet Based Tracking Programs and Software Apps

There are a number of websites and applications that will track your food intake and count your calories for you.

Lose It! (www.loseit.com) is one of the most popular and a wonderful tool for people with diabetes who want to lose weight. *The Greenwich Weight Loss and Diabetes Diet* is an independent publication and has not been authorized, sponsored, or otherwise approved by FitNow, Inc, doing business as Lose It! Feel free to use any program or app that works for you. There are also many sites that allow you to quickly calculate the calories in foods. Many of them allow you to enter information such as size or weight so that you get precise calories. Some popular ones are:

- www.dailyplate.com
- www.thecaloriecounter.com
- www.calorieking.com
- www.nutritiondata.com

Mobile Devices

Mobile devices have notes and word processing documents installed on them that can be used for your diary. For many people, mobile devices have replaced pens, papers, watches, and families.

WHEN AWAY FROM HOME

It was mentioned earlier that outings and vacations can prove to be a difficult time when it comes to keeping a food diary. We usually seek an escape from routines, responsibilities, and demands, and some of us consider our food diary a "chore". However, you still comb your hair and brush your teeth (hopefully) and perform other routine tasks while away from home, so consider your food diary as just another thing on your self-maintenance list. In reality, keeping your food diary requires nothing more than carrying paper and pen with you, and taking a whole 45 seconds to maintain your diary. Don't make more of it than it is.

THE POWER OF CALORIE COUNTING

Eating according to the SML carb guidelines will lower your blood sugar levels and help you lose weight. Once blood sugar levels stabilize over time, many of us hit a weight plateau, where we stop losing weight while sticking to the same diet. When this happens, the next step toward progress is to count calories. We're not going to discuss calories here, because there is more than enough information out there on the subject. Nevertheless, here are a few important points to consider:

A. Determine how many calories you are eating each day. Writing down the calories of the foods in your diary next to what you ate will increase your expertise in calorie counting. Don't go overboard and make it an onerous burden. Approximations will work and a quick pocket guide will do the trick. Of course, you can also find detailed information on calories on the websites or using one of the apps mentioned earlier.

B. One pound of body fat is about 3,500 calories. If you burn 500 calories more than you take in each day, you'll lose about a pound of fat a week. However, the actual amount you lose will also be influenced by your metabolic rate. Losing more than one pound each week is not recommended. There is often discomfort in the form of hunger and potential problems with blood sugar levels. If a 500-calorie decrease each day is too difficult, then try a 400-calorie deficit, or even a 300. In other words, go down in 100- calorie intervals until you find a tolerable intake level. It might take longer to lose weight, but give yourself credit for aiming in the right direction.

DETERMINE HOW MANY CALORIES YOU BURN EACH DAY

In order to best determine how many calories you burn each day, you'll want your metabolic rate determined. This is done professionally using a tool called an "indirect metabolic calorimeter". This kind of test requires you to sit for 15-30 minutes first thing in the morning with a device placed in your mouth. Your oxygen consumption and carbon dioxide production are measured to determine your resting metabolic rate (RMR). Your RMR is the amount of calories your body burns on a daily basis, not including physical activity. A distant second in accuracy is to determine your RMR by using a calculator, a number of which can be found online under a search for "RMR calculator". They are not great but can give you a rough idea of your RMR.

An alternative way to determine how many calories you burn each day, especially if you are physically active, is to use something called an "accelerometer". It is an armband or wrist watch-like device that fits on top or under your clothing. It tells you how many calories you burn each day. It measures every little movement you make. Some even let you know how many calories you are burning as you perform a specific activity. Some come with web-based programs, some provide live support coaches. They are usually compatible with the latest personal hand-held device.

Obviously, comparing the calories you take in with the calories you burn will give you concrete information you can use to adjust your caloric intake to ensure you lose weight. Measuring both caloric intake and output allows you to work at weight loss from both ends. If you've gotten to the lowest calorie intake with which you are comfortable, increase your exercises! You'll want to adjust the fuel consumed or the fuel burned, or both, if you want to lose weight.

EXTREME HUNGER MANAGEMENT

You may be one of us who swears we're following the SML food guidelines, but you still have periods during the day when you are so ravenously hungry, and you require superhuman willpower to avoid overeating. If you encounter this type of hunger in spite of following the SML guidelines, it is time to look for the origin of your extreme hunger. In order to fix it, you'll want to track down the specific cause. The good news is extreme hunger is fixable.

Tracking down the cause of excessive hunger usually means you'll want to take a second (or third) look at what you're eating, and then adjust your food intake. You can't do this without a food diary. Keep in mind your success is not measured by how rigidly you follow the recommended diet, regardless of how many gold stars you put on your food diary before you post it on your refrigerator door for all to see. Your success is measured by your ability to eat in a manner that allows you to comfortably avoid overeating and lose weight and enhance your quality of your life, the ultimate goal. If you can lose weight and be happy as well, you deserve a whole box of gold stars, and you can paste them on any darn thing you please!

If you are still having intense food cravings, you'll want to adjust parts of your SML intake. Understanding the SML basics gives you the tools required to fix the problem. At this point, you may feel like you hit a major obstacle, but now is not time to give up. You are just closer to succeeding. Now is the time to figure out what part of your new diet could be changed. Most often, the cause of your overeating is hidden in your food diary waiting to be discovered. You'll want to know how to look for the cause of the problem, how to recognize it when you see it, and finally, you'll want to know how to fix it. Sometimes the problems are all but jumping up and thumbing their noses at you. Upon discovery, you'll wonder what is wrong with you, that you didn't see the problem in the first place. Welcome to the club. Hey, we're new at this! In your quest to discover the cause of your extreme appetite, remember you are looking for the cause of the problem, and you are not on a mission to identify where you screwed up. Trial and error might be required until you find eating patterns and foods that work right for you. Remember, we're all a bit different, and how we react to various foods is different. The SML meal plan is like an off-the-rack suit. It has all the pieces: pants, jacket, and vest, and sure, it will fit some people without alterations, but in many cases, tailoring might be required for the proper fit. Please keep the following in mind:

- Extreme hunger may have a physiological or psychological (think "emotional") origin. If your hunger is emotionally based, tweaking your food intake is not going to help very much. Are you eating when you are anxious, sad, bored?

- We all react in our own way to different foods; so although you might know to which category an SML item belongs, the item may make your blood sugar levels spike differently than someone else's level.

- If you stabilize your blood sugar levels adequately through medications, exercise, and the right balance of SML carbs, you won't have unnatural, overwhelming, or uncontrollable cravings for food, either continuously or intermittently.

- If your meals are not sufficiently satisfying, your hunger will not be appeased, and it will act like a spoiled child and tantrum or pester you until you give in (it knows which techniques work best on you).

- Long-acting carbs are our stabilizers, so you want to be sure to eat enough of them. Many people are unaccustomed to eating lots of non-starch vegetables, so this is a common impediment and frequent solution to problems. Your food diary will reveal the amount of long-acting carbs you are actually eating.

- You can figure out why you are unusually hungry by looking at what types of carbs you previously ate before your extreme hunger and how long ago you ate them.

- You might want to experiment to find what works best, and give yourself time to adjust to those changes.

- To determine how your food choices affect your ravenous appetite, you may want to chart your satisfaction level after a meal and your hunger level throughout the day. Feel free to groan all you want upon hearing this. It is better than heading for the cookie jar!

- Not eating frequently enough can result in overeating that begins a vicious blood sugar rollercoaster. By now, you're well familiar with this whiplash inducing ride.

If the cause of your ruthless appetite is not emotionally based, but instead physiologically based, you'll want a plan of attack to identify the cause so you can fix it. Here are some steps you can take:

1. Your first step is to rule out being on a medication that causes an increase in appetite or affects your blood sugar level. Of course, don't discontinue or modify any medication without first talking to your doctor.

2. Monitor your blood sugar levels. It is ideal if one hour after your meal or snack your blood sugar level is no more than 40 points (mg/dl) higher that it was just before you ate. Two hours after your meal or snack, it is ideal if your blood sugar level is back where it was before you ate. Anything higher than this may indicate a spike high enough to trigger your ravenous appetite. If you can't address the blood sugar level increase by modifying your diet, you might want to talk to your doctor about changing your diabetes medications or discuss starting one if you are not on one.

3. Eating smaller portions and eating them more frequently often smooths out your blood sugar levels and helps avoid extreme spikes that lead to hunger. This can help prevent binge eating.

4. The cause of your extreme hunger is usually hidden in the details of your food diary. It can be well-camouflaged or obnoxiously obvious (just to taunt you).

5. If your meal is not satisfying or filling enough, you'll remain hungry. Consequently, you may want to modify your meal plan so you are both full and satisfied after a meal or snack. Charting your satisfaction level after a meal or snack on a scale of 1to 10 in a column added to your food diary, is an ideal way to help you see patterns and relationships between your food intake and your hunger. Stand back and try to look at the whole day. Hopefully you'll eventually be able to identify possible causes for your intense hunger and figure out how to

fix it. Be aware that you are looking for "adequate" or "acceptable" scores that indicate you are sufficiently satisfied. If you aim for nines and tens, you'll probably run into a problem. The trick is to feel "adequately" satisfied and to seek other non-eating ways to experience satisfaction.

6. Also on the same chart as your food diary, you can start noting your hunger level along with your satisfaction level. Waiting to eat until you are overly hungry can, and most likely will, result in overeating. Eating a little when you are a bit hungry can sometimes prevent you from overeating later. This is a common trap, because eating when we are less than extremely hungry seems to be contrary to our common sense and long-term practice. We're often used to fighting our hunger rather than work with it. Charting your hunger level hourly is ideal. You only have to do this until you find and fix the problem.

7. When you notice a major increase in your appetite, look back to see if your appetite can be accounted for in how you balanced your short-, medium-, and long-acting carbs during the meals and snacks preceding your exaggerated hunger. Remember, blood sugar spikes from short-acting carbs will start to decrease rapidly an hour or so after you consume them. If they fall from a high level, and you don't have medium- or long-acting carbs to soften their fall, you'll be very, very hungry! Remember, medium-acting carbs last longer and your blood sugar level will not decrease as quickly or as rapidly if they are in your system. Ask yourself: "Did I overdo the short-acting carb intake? Can I add more medium-acting or long acting-carbs?"

8. Notice the timing of your cravings. If your appetite surge comes within an hour or two after you eat, you may want to cut back on the short-acting carbs and/or increase the medium-and long-acting carbs. If you see many incidents of unusually intense cravings, you may want to increase the amount of long-acting carbs. Long-acting carbs are stabilizers. The balance between SML carbs are part of the tailoring you might want to do.

9. If you've had a day without intense hunger, study your food diary for that day. Try to understand why it worked for you.

You can compare your "hard days" to your "rough days" to help you understand how your food choices and when you eat influence your appetite.

10. Logging your food intake, satisfaction, and hunger levels, and then analyzing them is admittedly easier said than done, but it is certainly worth the effort. If you can't discover the cause of the problem or figure out how to fix it, you may benefit from working with an RD (registered nutritionist) familiar with the SML approach to eating. If you tried the above suggestions and don't have an RD available, there are workbooks that help you do this. One recommendation is Linda W. Craighead's book, *Appetite Awareness Workbook: How to Listen to Your Body and Overcome Bingeing, Overeating, and Obsession with Food.*

WINE FOR DESSERT?

There's no need to whine; you can have a glass or two of wine! Although drinking wine is not an approach to accelerate weight loss (it's just here for fun), a glass or two of wine might be a good replacement for desserts or snacks. Wine, especially red wine, has been touted for its cardiovascular health benefits and even anti-inflammatory and other properties. Researchers have also looked into how drinking wine affects those of us with diabetes. Drinking 1 or 2 glasses (not mugs, jugs, boxes, or tumblers!) of wine each day, considered moderate drinking, doesn't seem to have any negative effects on those of us with type-2 diabetes. In fact, some research suggests, but does not prove, that having a glass or two may actually be beneficial. The reason for the possible benefit probably has to do with alcohol lowering blood sugar, which in turn results in less insulin being secreted. This may lead to less sugar being stored away. If you already have a drink or two each day of something other than wine, you may want to consider switching to red wine (switching, not adding it to your intake) because it has very little sugar in it. Avoid beer; it is similar to having a slice of bread with each drink. Hard alcohol also has some of the benefits of wine, but due to the higher alcohol content in hard alcohol, it can sneak up on you and lead to hypoglycemia and binge eating, especially if you drink on an empty stomach. If you are not a drinker, there's not enough evidence to suggest it is beneficial for you to start drinking wine. Drinking more than a couple or three glasses a day at most is widely considered harmful.

HELP, I'VE STOPPED LOSING WEIGHT!

Weight loss can slow down or even appear to cease for some of us—even though we're sticking to our SLM meals and getting complements. If this happens to you, please be assured it is not payback for bragging about your weight loss…although the timing is often oddly suspicious. In some cases, you may still be losing weight, but perhaps not at a pace you're accustomed to. Then again, you may be losing weight, just not from areas of your body you are likely to notice. When your pace of weight loss becomes sluggish or stalls, you can once again blame your darn ancient ancestors. No doubt you inherited genes that trigger the release of hormones and other chemicals after you start losing weight. Your body perceives your weight loss as an indicator of famine. It now wants you to stop losing weight and actually prefers you even add on a few pounds for insurance. Frustrating? Absolutely! But you're too smart to fall for this biological trick of nature. You can outsmart your outdated body chemistry. You have the willingness and tools to work your way around this obstacle.

Don't be surprised if you become acutely aware of how tempted you are to deal with your frustration by eating. Not only could your increased appetite be a remnant from the past (eating to sooth your emotions), but your body may also be releasing hormones that signal you to eat more! Although the urge to eat may peak for you, your resilience and commitment are stronger forces, and you have new ways to deal with negative feelings. You can and will continue to lose weight as long as you stay true to your commitment to yourself and outsmart your biology. Just think of this slowdown as your fat trying to protect itself, because it knows it is unwanted and its days are numbered! Although it sure doesn't feel like it, it is a sign of weight loss success, not failure.

Once this biological famine switch is flipped, hormones begin racing through your body screaming "famine, famine, eat while you can"! This is your body's attempt to preserve its fat reserves. Your body might also start to use energy more efficiently by burning fewer calories at rest. This hoard of hormones and other biochemical survival mechanisms are all geared to increase your chance of survival (as if you're a cave dweller) by compelling you to eat more and conserve energy. To top it off, these changes are not usually temporary—they tend to stick around for a long time. Knowing this helps you weather the storm. Look at it this way:

The good news is:
You are an improved, more energy-efficient model of your former self.
The bad news is:
You are an improved, more energy-efficient model of your former self.

Just keep in mind you are still a lot better off than you were before your weight loss. Some people refer to this new more efficient model of yourself as your new metabolic "platform" or, alternatively as your new "set point" (think of it as a thermostat). For you, this is your new "normal." Weight gain or weight loss is now determined by how many extra calories you store or lose in comparison to your *new* set point. Although your pace of weight loss might not be as dramatic as it has been in the past, you can still continue to lose weight if you pledge allegiance to your long-term goals, and remember you're in it for the long haul.

Fortunately, there's something you can do to offset this slowdown: readjust your set point. There's only one way to reset your body's metabolic set point: exercise! Exercise increases your metabolism (which helps burn fat), decreases your sugar level, makes you physically stronger, and leads to overall better health. It is an excellent way to accelerate weigh loss!

✸   ✸   ✸

Chapter 10

OH NO, NOT EXERCISE!

So, maybe not all of us have a hard time exercising or starting an exercise program. We may want a bit of encouragement, a few practical tips, perhaps some non-edible reward, and we're good to go. However, a rather large number of us find the thought of exercising so unpleasant we'd prefer to skip this chapter altogether. In fact, some of us are so extreme in our fear or dislike of exercise that we're already hatching a plan to avoid it. We might even tell ourselves we'll start exercising after we lose some weight and feel more comfortable. Although there are solid tips here that will help you regardless of your level of resistance to exercise or amount of weight you want to lose, this chapter is geared more toward those of us having the most difficulties with exercising. It seems that the larger we are, the harder it is to embrace exercising (or more accurately, tolerate it). Some of us (how tempting to name names), joke that we are "allergic" to exercise. It is a good way to change the subject and avoid the seriousness of our problem.

Exercise is important because it not only burns calories and fat, but is also a great weight loss maintainer. Our bodies have a built in "set point" for weight that it tries to maintain. A set point is like an automatic thermostat to maintain a certain weight. If we lose weight, our body will urge us to overeat to get back to the set point. Exercise appears to reset our set-point. It could be that the pleasure experienced after exercise (not during it) might replace some of the satisfaction we derived from eating. No one knows how it works, but regardless, it works! This is an added benefit. Exercise burns calories, enhances our metabolism, and can provide us a sense of accomplishment. It's like a three-for-one special. How could you resist?

I'd Like to Exercise, But…

There is something about exercise and excess weight that just doesn't fit well together. It feels like an arranged marriage. The more you weigh, the faster you are probably tempted to skim this chapter. For some of us, exercise is the last thing in the world we want to do, and if we list "have a beautiful, fit, and sexy body" on our bucket list, we're referring to being with someone who fits that description, not attaining that goal ourselves. We wish we liked to exercise, but we simply don't. We tried it; we didn't like it. Sure, we know that it increases our metabolism, empowers us, and is good for both our mind and body. Knowing these things, however, just isn't enough to change our attitude or behavior. Besides, we tell ourselves exercise has taken on a whole new meaning since we were young. We didn't even call our physical activities exercise, we called it play, and the playful activity was natural, usually unplanned, and downright fun. Back then, we were only out to have fun; physical activity (now called exercise) was just a means to an end, not an end in itself. Perhaps this is why it seems so alien to many of us.

There Are No Amish gyms!

Exercise, as we now usually think of it, is a rather modern invention. Up until the last few generations, we didn't go out of our way to exercise; we didn't have to plan or schedule it in. People got their exercise naturally, without expensive equipment and special locations such as gyms to conduct this bizarre, unnatural activity. Attending a good, strenuous hoedown, or going to a barn raising, now that's natural exercise! You want an upper body workout? Try baling hay or churning butter for crying out loud! However, exercise, as unnatural as it now seems, grows out of the desire to counterbalance the way we live (and eat) these days. No wonder it feels like punishment; it really is payback for participating in "the good life"! We want the benefits of modern society without the liabilities; there's nothing wrong with that…until you realize the consequences. But until we can come up with much better pills, or join some religious group or cult that rejects the conveniences of modern society, planned exercise is here to stay. If you don't have a problem with exercising, and have incorporated a healthy exercise program into your lifestyle, congratulations! There are a lot of us very jealous of you. Unless you want to learn about how the "other half lives," you may want to spend your time exercising rather than reading the rest of this chapter (or better, just scan the headings). But for the rest of us, perhaps the majority of us, want to figure out how to make the best of our situation. It would be nice if we think of exercise as we do toothbrushing—just doing it as part of our daily routine. We can do that.

Raising Awareness

Those who don't carry around substantial excess weight might not fully appreciate how unappealing exercising can be for us. They haven't "walked the walk," so how could we expect them to fully appreciate how we feel? That's why it is our job, our moral responsibility, to sensitize them by strapping a couple ten-pound bags of sugar onto their hips. At the end of the day, have them bend over, remove their shoes while standing, and then ask them how they feel! Sadly, some of us would be happy to carry only two, ten-pound bags on our hips. The harsh reality is that many of us carry around the equivalent of much more than a couple ten-pound bags of sugar, and we've done it for many years.

If polled, most of us who are significantly overweight would say we are not against exercising, we're just against *us* exercising! The extremists among us would even admit we liken exercise to punishment for being fat. Of course, we know that it isn't, but we just can't shake that idea. We think we have to exercise because we're fat, when in fact it would be sensible to exercise even if we weren't overweight. If you feel negatively about exercising, you are not alone. Knowing you aren't alone is always comforting, but it doesn't provide solutions. If we knew how to solve this problem, we would. We're not stupid… and we're not lazy! So, what's with us? Why are we struggling, and how are we different from those who seem to have no problem exercising regularly?

So, What's Wrong with Me?

Many people exercise regularly knowing they are doing something good for their body. They take pride in their body, and even the little bit of physical discomfort they experience reminds them that they are successfully meeting their goals. They experience satisfaction knowing they master the task at hand. Rumor has it that some people—sit down for this one—actually set their alarms so they can get up early and exercise *before* they go to work! Honestly, you just can't make this stuff up! So why can't we tap into some of that "mojo"? What's wrong with us or right with them? Where can we find some of the enthusiasm and motivation they possess? Why are we fighting the mere idea of exercising, or in an extreme, avoiding it at all cost? Good grief, we can break into a sweat just thinking about exercising!

If the above rant fires you up, or you feel it speaks for you even a little, it was a bit of a snare, a trap…a cheap trick! It demonstrates how vulnerable you (as well as many others of us) are to buying into a negative view about exercise. It is easy to convince people to hate exercise. If the dislike is not already apparent, it is often just below the surface. However, hold on to those negative feelings and terrible images of exercise for a while. You'll find they provide a good contrast to some other points of view, and will help you put the mere idea of exercising into perspective.

Is Our Attitude Just a Frame of Reference?

Sure, we have a very different attitude than those who get up very early in the morning to exercise, but there's another group that also provides a good contrast: Flashback: 1968, tie-dye, Chicago, Eunice Kennedy Shriver's six years of summer camps for people with developmental disabilities results in the first Special Olympics. Folks with developmental disabilities have their first official physical competition. The thrill of competing, the pride of physical achievement, and the outcome of hours of practice is finally paying off! Just having the opportunity to compete makes them an instant winner! The laughter, smiles, and jumps of joy over personal achievements are no less genuine than they are for any other person competing in any other type of physical sport. All participants are winners, and being a winner takes absolutely nothing away from the achievement of other individual winners! All the ribbons are equally appreciated, all pats on the back equally meaningful, and all the joy of accomplishment equally sincere. Sure the applause of the crowd helps, but we can provide our own applause if desired. Their ability to experience the satisfaction of mastery is not due to their disabilities, it is there in spite of them. It comes from a different frame of reference than ours, a different standard for achievement. It is a personal achievement because it meets personal expectations. They did not and still do not spend their time moping and complaining their Olympics it not the *real* Olympics they see on TV. That's not the point. Everyone who shows up and tries their best is a winner. Why can't *we* do the same? Why can't *you* do the same? Our acceptance or rejection of exercise is about personal expectations, attitudes, and equally if not more important, appreciating our personal achievements. Set your own bar. Doing so can change the way you think about exercise. What thoughts and ideas currently pop into your head when you think of exercise? Are they the negative ones mentioned earlier? What thoughts and ideas would work better for you? Both those participating in the Special Olympics and those early morning go-getters have a different frame of reference than we do, and there is no reason we can't have a positive one too.

By changing our thinking, we make it easier to lose weight and change our bodies. When the negative thoughts about exercise pop up, replace them with your new frame of reference. You may feel a bit silly doing this at first, but you'll feel differently after you see that it works. Replace the "I hate exercise" frame and idea with, "I want to lose weight and feel better about myself." Be sure to set it up so you are guaranteed to win your own ribbon and experience pride.

Don't Exercise!

We all exercise from the moment our feet hit the floor. We call it moving. Yet, when thinking of exercise, most of us fall into the trap of visualizing rather unattractive situations, such as: excessive effort, physical discomfort, sweat and odor, skin irritations, uncomfortable heart rates, unattractive appearances, unflattering clothing, etc. Before you can tackle true cardio-vascular, aerobic or other forms of formal exercising, it makes sense to ease into it. Set it up so you win. If you're having a hard time jumping into a structured exercise program, first simply think about increasing your movement—natural movement—the type of movement that was once considered normal. This physical movement will feel more natural and less contrived. Think of it as increasing your activity level rather than "exercise" if that helps.

Instead of an "exercise plan," try developing a "movement plan"— a conscious effort to comfortably increase the extent and duration of your physical movements throughout the day. Invest that physical energy doing activities that are fulfilling and not isolated from life's normal activities. It is highly suggested you find an activity that is enjoyable, or better, one that offers additional rewards outside of the physical activity itself. Of course, you'll check with your doctor(s) to determine if there are any physical limitations on exercising.

Examples:

1. Walking: If you are usually bombarded by stimuli and demands, you probably want your daily dose of "freedom." A daily walk could be your escape. It serves two purposes, and this certainly makes it more attractive. The "freedom" might feel so refreshing that you find yourself extending the length of time you walk, not to get more exercise, but to get more freedom time. If it has been an aggravating day, you might find yourself increasing your pace as a way of "letting go" of some of the tension that has built up. Some people find their attention naturally drift when they walk, and others spend the walk time problem solving and thinking things through, an activity easier done with fewer distractions. If you start walking, you will find your own form of freedom. Headphones (or ear-buds) can supply music, an audio-book, etc. Besides, you'll get less lip if you say you want to get your "exercise in" than you would if you say, "I want some me time." You are encouraged to create and take ample "me time".

2. Dancing: You have many types from which to choose, and the thought of dancing puts smiles on many faces. If you've ever said, "I wish I could dance like that," start looking for opportunities. Square dancing anyone? Zumba? Ballroom? Just choose one that will make you smile! Be sure to double check the health status of your joints, as you do not want to cause harm. Some forms of dance and exercise can be very rough on joints.

3. Friend's Choice: Pick your best friend's favorite activity. Hang out and move together. You'll be so involved in the latest gossip, sport, or get-rich-quick scheme you'll forget you are also doing it for your body!

4. Swimming: How wonderful for heavy people to feel weightless! The only problem is that you might not want to get out. Taking pressure off our joints is an additional bonus for many of us, although your shoulders might get more of a workout than you want. Check out water aerobics, too!

5. Bicycling: This is kind of like walking with support and with the wind in your face. You can even coast! If you enjoyed it as a kid, you can enjoy it now…if you let yourself!

THE TEN BARRIERS TO EXERCISE

Of course, not all readers have the same degree of resistance, or the same type of resistance. Others don't understand what this big fuss is about and why there is even a need for this chapter. They call us whiners behind our backs. They should hear what we call them! The following recommendations are for everyone, but those of us who find it harder to add regular exercise to our lifestyle might find the list of the top barriers especially helpful. The list of the top ten barriers to exercise, along with some possible solutions, are:

Barrier 1: I have no time to exercise.

Make time. Don't take this the wrong way, but we've received anonymous notes telling us you engage in the following activities:

A. You occasionally hit the snooze button to get an extra 10 minutes of sleep. On more than one occasion (we have the dates if you're interested), you've hit more than once!
B. You are occasionally seen sauntering over to the vending machine, stopping to chat along the way. Your discussions don't really sound like work-related conversations unless you're either a sports announcer or local news reporter. The last observation clocked your little "summit" as lasting 12 minutes and 18 seconds…approximately.
C. Okay, checking email is important, but most of your friends agree you can eliminate one of the 10-minute, daily sessions, and not lose contact. Besides, you occasionally forward the same joke more than once. This is unnecessary. Your friends are pleading!

It is not comfortable putting you on the spot, but if you add up the above minutes, this equals the amount of time it would take you to complete a 30-minute walk (plus 2 minutes and 18 seconds to change your shoes). Some of the busiest and most important people in the world make time for physical activity (they no doubt call it "my workout"). You may believe you don't have time, but it may be a misperception, or, possibly, you don't know how to create the time you want. Don't confuse the two.

Don't get caught up thinking that you have to exercise for a long duration in order to achieve benefits. Also, don't take seriously the recommendations such as you "should" complete "at least 20 minutes of cardiovascular exercise 5 days a week." In fact, some gurus would have you training 7 days a week and 90 minutes each day, and even demand strength training along with your cardiovascular workout. By aiming high, they are not quite saying that anything less than their recommendation is useless. In fact, several studies show that just a few minutes a week can lead to improved metabolic functioning. How few? Just 7 minutes a day makes all the difference!

Don't set up barriers; start modestly. Once you are exercising for 7 minutes, if you don't feel better after giving it a fair shot, stop at 7 minutes. In some cases, we are all but "rehabbing" ourselves (if you can get into a rehab program, go for it!), and want to approach accomplishments in small increments. If you are unable to meet your set goal, you set your goal too high. Beg yourself for forgiveness and make the necessary correction.

Barrier 2: Getting started and restarted.

You are usually in the greatest discomfort at the beginning of an exercise, and then it eases up. The discomfort is more mental than physical. As you continue your exercise, the middle starts becoming more uncomfortable again, yet something special usually happens: Although uncomfortable, you believe the goal is in site, and when you feel you're approaching it, you feel pleasure. Often, this pleasure compels you to "push it" until things become so painful you're forced to stop. Here's a secret: don't push to failure! If you end your activity in pain, your brain will remember the extreme discomfort of the final push and you'll have a big mental barrier in your head the next time you go to exercise. This is one reason many of us dislike the idea of exercising, yet we can't figure out why. Instead, it is better to end the exercise session when we are minimally uncomfortable. Although you don't have to "push it" when exercising, if you do "push it" be sure to "cool down" after the "push". Cooling down is essential for both physiological as well as psychological reasons. You'll have better memories of the workout and will therefore be more likely to exercise next time. Remember: Your next workout begins the way your last one ended. If you end in pain, there will be a big mental barrier next time.

Barrier 3: Ouch, it hurts!

You don't want exercise to be painful. Exercise can be done at a pace and rhythm you can sustain for a reasonable period of time. Forget the old adage "no pain, no gain". It isn't true, and it is counterproductive. Pain associated with exercise can be debilitating. Pain and injury decreases exercise, sometimes stopping it. Because of this, losing weight can come to an end, or worse, weight gain can occur. Consequently, your body will be in poorer shape because of it. This type of situation can lead to a downward spiral. It is no exaggeration or scare tactic to say that this downward spiral can result in you ending up in a wheelchair. The sad thing is that in many cases, this scenario is avoidable. Once in a wheelchair, you'd pray for the opportunity to walk 30 minutes a day, and would be pleased to do so in the worst of weather and in pain. Everything is relative. When you look for excuses to avoid exercising, think of those individuals who can't. This isn't a low down, dirty, cheap, tasteless trick; it allows you to see things in a new manner with a heavy dose of reality on the side.

When the weight starts coming off, you'll be able to do more exercise with less effort. Success breeds success, but you want to give yourself the opportunity to experience success. Let yourself get caught up in it, get swirling in your own self-created upward spiral. You can do it. It is within everyone's reach.

Barrier 4: I don't know what exercise to do!

Here's a beauty, a real gem of advice: "Move in a way that makes you smile." Darn, that could have been the name of this chapter! Once you get the okay from your doctor to exercise (get specifics from him or her, cover all major body parts and joints), think about any movement that makes you smile—be it walking, swimming, dancing, roller skating, or chasing squirrels. As long as you are safe and you are smiling, keep on going!

People often argue over what type of exercise is "best" for diabetes control and weight loss. The truth is they're all good. The most popular and effective, however, appears to be walking. It's probably not for the reasons that you think. Sure, walking improves circulation, and burns calories and fat, but it also supports all of your body weight, has a low chance of injury, does not depend on a facility, and does not crash your blood sugars.

Walking

When you walk without using any physical aids or appliances (such as walkers, crutches, treadmill arms, or shopping carts), you support your whole body. When you support your entire bodyweight during exercise, you expend much more energy than if holding onto or sitting on something. The beauty of walking is that your body does not recognize how much extra energy is being burned. How many calories you actually burn depends on a number of things: your height, weight, overall condition, and unique body chemistry. When comparing exercises, you'll want to consider your discomfort level. If you don't, you might be comparing apples to oranges. For example, a man with huge deltoids would perceive his effort to swim to be less than someone without huge deltoids. Also, peddling a bike on a flat terrain for 10 miles is not the same as peddling uphill the same distance. Be aware of generic calculators that estimate the number of calories burned; they don't usually take discomfort level into consideration. The effort put into exercising must be equal across all the forms of exercise in order to make fair comparisons. Let's look at Mr. Smith, and pretend his effort level, time spent, and discomfort level are all equal. This is how his various options might compare:

A. If walking at 2 mph, he will burn about 35 calories.

B. If he swims at 1 mph, he'll burn about 25 calories, because water is supporting some of his body weight.

C. If he cycles at about 10 mph, he will burn about 30 calories (a stationary bike is about the same if it has the same discomfort level). This is because he is sitting and holding onto handles to support his weight, not to mention the kinetic energy of the bicycle (an object in motion stays in motion…). Remember, the amount of resistance must equal the same discomfort level of the other exercises.

D. The calories he would burn chasing squirrels have not been determined.

There are a number of other advantages of walking compared to some other sports:

A. We're experienced at it. Unless you've been carried around much of your life in a sedan chair by servants, you won't have to learn a new skill. Your chances of falling are minimal compared to other exercises like cycling or rollerblading.

B. The workload is dispersed when walking. Because we use our entire lower body to walk, many muscles, bones, and tendons share the load. This is not always the case with other exercises or activities such as swimming.

C. Walking creates less impact on our bones and joints than many other activities. This decreases the odds of becoming injured.

D. Walking typically does not lead to a crash of our blood glucose levels, as some other types of exercises can do. Our body likes to use two types of fuel during exercise, fat, and sugar. It might also use protein from muscle if really starved for energy, but this is unlikely.

Barrier 5: I hate gyms!

You are not alone if you hate gyms. Many of us heavier people would have to be physically forced to enter one. So, if you're as indignant as many of us, where do you go to exercise? First, figure out what exercise makes you smile, then find a local path, dance class, roller rink, trail, or court, enlist a walking partner, etc. and get going. Think "old fashioned" and figure out where the more natural locations are for the activity that makes you smile. If it requires special clothing (with the exception of shoes for clog dancing or a harness for trapeze) it might make it easier for you to get started if you don't require "gear". Getting involved in learning a new set of skills could work against or for you. If it is something you wanted to learn to do, and it is motivating, and you get exercise from the onset, go for it! If it is going to take training and/ or practice just to get to the point of enjoying it or getting a decent amount of exercise from it, move on to another option…briskly.

Enlisting the assistance of a gym or personal trainer is not to be dismissed, because it would be unfair to discourage anyone from getting this extra help if they are motivated by this; however, relying upon one for your daily exercise is usually a mistake. To get into a daily routine, we do best with the fewest obstacles possible. There is a lot to be said for "standing on your own two feet," and it is even better when, once standing, you start walking. Here's why a gym might be a mistake, especially for a beginner:

A. Some of us are too self-conscious or embarrassed to be seen in a gym, and going to a gym would create a bad experience and therefore lessen the chance we will return.

B. They have limited hours and are closed for holidays.

C. It takes more planning and effort to get to a gym than some other possible locations. The more steps involved, the greater the chance there will be a problem. Having to drive to a gym and deal with weather and parking is simply not attractive (unless your household is so chaotic that you find blizzards or hurricanes a step toward tranquility).

D. Gyms can become crowded during certain times of the day, often when you too want to use it.

E. The equipment you want to use might be occupied, and prying bodybuilders off equipment can be too strenuous even if you use mace.

F. There are machines with weight limits! Ugh…what were they thinking? What could be worse than being approached and questioned about your weight?

G. Many of us are not comfortable with our weight and body. Yelling out, "Quit staring at me," every few minutes sometimes backfires and draws even more unwanted attention. Besides, it just adds another thing to your "to do" list.

Be creative. There's the great story of a rather large man who wanted to swim (because it made him smile) who was too self-conscious of his weight to use the local public pool. Unfortunately, he didn't own a pool himself. He placed an ad offering to clean someone's pool if they let him swim in it during the day when they were at work. He had many offers from which to choose, and chose to be "adopted" by the owner of an indoor pool, which allowed him to swim all year long.

Barrier 6: I can't get into a routine!

Setting up a realistic routine for daily exercise can be difficult. It often relies on choosing a time of day when you are least likely to be distracted. For most of us, this time is the morning, but it can be at any time during the day. One disadvantage of mornings, however, is that when you are in bed, just prior to rising, your brain operates not unlike that of a three-year-old child, and not a particularly gifted child at that. If a three year old would have trouble doing something, you will too. Think about what would give a three year old trouble: picking out clothes, making a cup of coffee, pouring cereal, figuring out what walking route to take, etc. The only way around this is to prepare everything you require in the morning *before* you retire for the night. Stumbling around preparing things before bed is still better than having to cope with an all but dysfunctional brain in the morning. Your wake up, preparation, and walking route requires being so unencumbered that a three year old could follow it. You'll want the coffee to be ready to go with a touch of the switch, or better yet, be on a timer. It is best if your clothing is both close and appropriate for the activity (e.g., extremely warm clothes for walking). Breakfast and medications can all be placed on the table, and refrigerated breakfast items at the front of the shelf. Remember, upon first awakening, even the smallest hindrance can sabotage your best plans, and your three-year-old brain is looking for any flimsy excuse it can to hit the snooze button, which you may want to affectionately rename the "exercise derail button".

Barrier 7: I'm afraid of hypoglycemia if I exercise!

Strenuous exercises such as weight training are very beneficial for both diabetes and weight control, and yes, they must be approached cautiously. They lower blood sugar; burn significant calories, increases fitness, increases metabolism, etc. However, they can diminish blood sugar significantly, and if those of us with diabetes are unaware of this, strenuous exercise might sometimes lead to hypoglycemia (low blood sugar). Hypoglycemia is unpleasant, but when it occurs as a result of exercise, it can be a binge "wild card". This is to say the consequence can't be predicted. It could either result in nausea or extreme cravings. There is no way to predict what course it will take. If you get hit with cravings, you'll desire "decadent" foods. When this happens, odds are that you are going to consume far more calories than you just burned…way more. One step forward, two steps back? Not a good strategy.

Always play safe by keeping glucose tablets around. Many of us feel so good immediately after exercising that we don't want to undermine our achievement by eating; we're on a good roll and don't want it to end. Chances are, however, once the high ends, you'll be feasting and consuming more as a result of the postponement, so be careful. Also, waiting too long to eat after exercise may decrease your recovery rate and as well as fitness gain.

Barrier 8: I won't do things I "have" to do!

It is common reaction to want to push back or hold your ground when you hear demands such as, "have to," "must," or "should". The truth is you don't have to do a darn thing; no one is making you do anything. Well, no one but you, that is. It is your own internal dialogue. If you are going to argue with yourself ("I should/I won't"), it will result in a standoff. Standoffs can go on for years, no… decades…. no, lifetimes.

Even though we might realize that we feel better when we exercise, many of us distort things, and tell ourselves exercise will not be pleasurable. It is difficult to break away from this type of thinking. First, you have to admit that your brain is not perfect and didn't come with an instruction manual (much less a maintenance schedule). You might be helped in your struggle if you know that many people are trapped by expecting bad outcomes or lack of pleasure when they think of future events. It is a mindset, a very harmful one. One common example is forcing yourself to attend an event, only to later admit to yourself, "Boy, I'm glad I went"! When the next similar event occurs, you go through the same thing, sometimes even recognizing your poor predicting ability as a bit of a pattern. This is because some of us have a poor ability to predict pleasurable outcomes (poor pleasure prediction or PPP). Despite our experience and memory, our brain is telling us that we'll be in more pain and will feel worse if we exercise. Don't buy into this. It is faulty reasoning, and you have the wherewithal to recognize it as such. You can remind yourself that you are a poor predictor of pleasure and discard those poor predictions. Just think of it being one of your "quirks" and toss those negative predictions aside.

You will also benefit by creating plans with as few mental and physical barriers as possible. The big mental barriers are: "I have to, need to, must exercise." It is odd, but those of us saddled with nagging "shoulds" also know, on another level, we want to exercise. If you can't erase the "I must, should, need to…" out of your mind, then add to the thought by completing the sentence with, "but I *want* to, because I would *like* to lose weight, decrease my anxiety, have more energy, stabilize my blood sugar…" Move past the "shoulds" and get in touch with what you really want. Give your wants a stronger voice. Standoffs only end when one party becomes better armed, stronger or outsmarts the other.

Don't set yourself up for any big hurdles. Start small, very, very, small if you want. Set 100% guaranteed, achievable goals. Give yourself a ribbon just for showing up. Sure you'll tell yourself, "That was easy, anyone could have done that!" But that's just being critical. Knock it off! Your brain will know better, and nothing breeds success like success, even small successes. You'll find yourself expecting a bit more of yourself, and slowly you will adopt a more positive attitude.

It is kind of like outsmarting your brain. Remember, if an exercise doesn't make you smile, find another exercise!

Barrier 9: I get enough exercise already!

A frequent protest is, "I'm running around the house, up and down the stairs, chauffeuring kids around, and hauling groceries, so certainly I'm getting enough exercise…yet, I'm still fat!" First, it is wonderful that you are so active! Consider yourself a step ahead of many of us. But there is no reason why an active individual can't benefit by adding more planned movement to their day. Take time for yourself that is not part of taking care of others or related to "chores". It is good not only for your physical health, but also your mental health. If you are already in good shape, why not get in better shape? Remember to find an exercise that makes you smile. It is unlikely the "running around" you are currently doing is making you smile, even if you are generally a cheerful person.

Barrier 10: I'm sorry, but I simply can't motivate myself to exercise.

Sometimes even the best suggestions don't fit, because they don't address the real problem. If you can't get over the humps, and simply can't even begin a modest form of exercise, you may be too depressed. Many seriously depressed people are simply unable to get to the point of exercising without first getting some help. There is a reason you can't get going, and help is available. Here are three things to think about:

1. Self-criticism is the greatest de-motivator.

2. Treat yourself no less than you would someone you admire.

3. If knowing the above is not helpful to you, you might be seriously depressed.

HOW TO SWEETEN YOUR REWARD

Ideally, we all want to be attuned to how our health affects (or will later affect) others, such as family and friends. In this way, we are increasing our motivation. Knowing you are putting effort into something that will not only pay off for you, but also for your family and loved ones, might help you get going. This is not asking you to con-sider "guilt" as a motivator for exercising, but to recognize that others might benefit from your actions. Guilt might get you started, but it won't hold up as well as a long-term motivator. It is better to approach exercise more positively. But even knowing how family or loved ones might benefit may still fall short of getting some of us motivated to exercise. There is also one more thing all of us might want to consider, whether or not we lack motivation. And that is to combine our exer-cise with activities that help others.

We're all formed from different dough (or Silly Putty in some cases) and some of us simply do a better job caring for others than we do caring for ourselves. If you are one of the special people cut from the "helper" cookie cutter, consider getting your exercise by helping someone or something else. There are puppies and dogs that will give you unconditional love if you take them for a walk. There are many dogs in small cages either sitting or standing on concrete, waiting for the slightest bit of attention. They would delight in the freedom to be in fresh air and exercise for a half hour once in a while. Their enthu-siasm is contagious, their excitement distracting, and their influence upon us unique and unquestionably positive. There are also home-bound individuals who find it difficult or impossible to walk their dog, and in many cases, the dog is the most important living thing in their life. The dog *and* the owner would both welcome you with open paws and arms. It probably wouldn't even feel like exercise! Sometimes the need for help is permanent, and sometimes temporary, such as some-one recovering from an accident or surgery. Imagine trying to walk your dog during chemotherapy. Boarding kennels, veterinarians, homecare services, and religious centers are all good contacts. There are others.

Similarly, for many of the same reasons, many people can't get out to do their own shopping, especially grocery shopping. If you are feeling down, grumpy, dissatisfied or unenthusiastic, focusing on someone else's needs might be the first step toward respecting and appreciating your own. If you go to the grocery store for someone, be aware that pushing a cart is a bit easier than walking. You might want to push the cart around, empty or loaded, non-stop for a given amount of time before circling around to pick up the items actually on your list. You'll even get a little upper body workout by lifting the groceries. If you desire, you can set up a point system by allotting yourself predetermined points depending upon the size display you knock over each trip. Keep written records. Your local department for the aging, religious institutions, visiting nurse service, homecare providers, and others can help you get started. If they tell you their client list is confidential, ask them to pass your number to the person in need. Call around until you get someone who appreciates your generous offer and is willing to take a few minutes to call their clients. Just one warning: keep it manageable, offer small, time-limited commitments you know you can fulfill. You can always extend your time, but avoid unintentionally setting up dependency relationships that could end in feelings of abandonment...hey; this is supposed to be a feel good thing! Knowing a person or a dog needs you, wants you, and is expecting you, is sometimes just the motivation helpful to get you going. If you stop to think about it, there are other things you can do that benefit others and your community and that also benefits you physically. It's like the old days when people helped each other.

GO UNNATURAL AND HIGH-TECH!

Okay, so this is a total switch from much of the above, but this might be a solution for some. You say you'd rather play than exercise? Then treat yourself to a wireless video-game console. You can participate in sports, excursions, games, dances, and other physical activities right in front of the TV. People in nursing homes are tripping over each other to ensure they are the first in line when staff turns on the console. You wouldn't believe the language that comes out of their mouths as they race to cue up! How fitting that the problems caused by living in our "modern" society might just be addressed by high technology.

TIPS FOR THE PHYSICALLY CHALLENGED AND DISABLED

Not all of us are fully able to participate in some of the exercises mentioned. This does not mean you can't exercise, it just means that you exercise within your particular requirements, strengths, and limitations. Talk to your physician, and if you want, see if you can consult with a physical therapist, sports medicine physician, or rehabilitation specialist. They can help set you up with an individualized exercise program.

A great start for individuals with cardiac or respiratory problems is a cardio-pulmonary rehab program. They are outstanding and improve overall quality of life.

Individuals unable to fully use their lower limbs will find some interesting videos on the Internet under searches for: "wheelchair exercises," "adaptive exercises," or "exercise for the disabled". If you visit www.youtube.com you'll find instructional videos of all types. If you search around, or have someone search for you, you will find help for those of us also dealing with sensory impairments. Go for it!

EXERCISE AND WEIGHT LOSS

Exercise burns our body's fuels and results in weight loss. Fat breaks down about 3 times as fast when exercising than when we are at rest. In general, we burn fats and carbs in the form of sugars during exercise. Of course, how much we burn depends on our nutrition, the shape we're in, and the type of exercise we're doing and the duration of the exercise. Here are a few things to keep in mind:

1. If your blood sugar level is high, exercise will immediately start to burn off the excess sugar. If you blood sugar is extremely high, such as over 350, exercise won't help and might make matters worse.

2. If we exercise for long periods, we will burn fat along with some sugars.

3. High intensity exercises, such as sprinting, jumping, weight lifting and throwing use more blood sugar. Monitor your blood sugar level carefully if you're engaging in intense exercises.

4. Protein plays a minor role when exercising, but eating an adequate amount of protein is critical for maintaining muscle mass.

5. During the first 20-30 minutes of intense exercise, we burn primarily blood sugar as well as sugar stored in our muscles (called glycogen) and a small amount of fat for energy. At about the 20-30-minute mark, however, our body begins to utilize a higher percentage of body fat for energy and a

lesser percentage of glucose. This is often called the "fat burning zone," because fat is our primary source of fuel after the 30-minute mark.

EATING, DRINKING, AND EXERCISE

First, remember to stay well hydrated at all times. If you engage in strenuous exercise, it is important to eat properly before and after exercising. You'll want to ensure a proper mix of short-acting carbs (simple carbs), fat, and protein. The simple carbs will provide energy, fats will provide sustainability, and protein is for muscle health. It is best if you eat anywhere between 30 and 90 minutes before exercising and eat short-acting carbs, protein and some fat again immediately after you exercise. For mild to moderate exercise, eating before or immediately after exercising is not recommended.

COOLING DOWN AND STRETCHING

Don't forget to properly stretch and cool down when exercising. You don't want to stretch cold muscles. Instead stretch them after they are warmed. The goal of stretching is to warm your muscles with the goal of increasing their flexibility, blood flow to your muscles, and your range of motion, all of which help prevent injuries. Don't forget to "cool down" for at least the last 5 minutes of your exercise. The cool down is better if it is gradual and decreases in intensity. Both techniques help regulate your blood flow and limit or control dizziness.

Certainly, exercise will help you control your blood sugar and help you lose weight. Diabetes is a physical disease, but who would ever imagine that how you think can influence your blood sugar and weight? Think your way to thinness? You must be kidding!

✲ ✲ ✲

Chapter 11

CONTROL YOUR BLOOD SUGAR AND WEIGHT WITH YOUR MIND!

It is nothing less than amazing to learn that we can control our blood sugar levels and weight by the way we think. What's even more remarkable is that our thoughts and mental state affect us in not one, but two different ways:

1. Our thoughts trigger feelings that trigger our behaviors, including eating behavior.

2. Anxiety and depression can cause changes in our body chemistry that directly affect our blood sugar levels. We'll get to this mind-altering discussion later.

THOUGHTS

When awake, we are constantly thinking (unless perhaps we are in a deep meditative state). Most of our thoughts seem to be automatic. One thought leads to another in an unending, loosely connected series like links in a chain, sometimes called a "stream of thought." Some thoughts are intentional, purposeful and directed, such as balancing our financial accounts (which is often followed by weeping). Other thoughts seem to just pop up, something akin to daydreaming, but not the kind of daydreaming you do about spending your lottery winnings—that's purposeful thinking, planning. Instead, the form of daydreaming being referred to is that "silly" (ouch, how judgmental!) thinking that seems to roam on its own and jump from one thought to another connected by a thin, sometimes even invisible thread. We have about 50,000 of these automatic thoughts each day. No wonder we need to sleep! Here's an example of a stream of thought:

My feet hurt.
I need to cut my toenails.

My clippers are probably in the top drawer of my desk.
I really shouldn't keep them there, that's nasty!
Clippers? Yes, that reminds me I need go to the drugstore.
I wonder if that new medication is a tier 2 or 3 price level.
Ugh, I'll wait until I pick it up to find out; I hate talking to people on the phone.
Actually, a lot of people seem to annoy me. Why are so many people annoying?
Maybe it is just me. There aren't that many people who I really like.
That Mary Ann is really an exception, I like her. She's a keeper.
Mary is the name of my niece, too.
I can't think of little Mary without thinking of when she threw up on me years ago.
I sure did a good job acting as if I was cool with it.
She sure is a mess now, drugs and all. How did this all happen?
Ugh, thinking about her makes my stomach clench, I feel so sad for sis.
Maybe a nice cup of tea would be soothing right now.
No, not just tea, I need to stop and enjoy life for a few minutes, so I'll have some cookies, too.
There's nothing like real British tea made the right way.
I really like the British. Rule Britannia!
What's better, to say English or British? I don't really care. Why do I worry about such things?
I'm so stupid sometimes.
The royal family is always in the news; I couldn't live like that if I were a member.
That Camilla is having the last laugh, isn't she?
She must be interesting to talk to and probably has really good gossip!
I wonder if she cuts her own toenails.
No, of course not, that was a stupid thought!
I need to cut my toenails.
Umm, well maybe after a cup of tea…and cookies.

Now, the above is not the best example of a wandering mind, because it doesn't include thoughts of a sexual nature, unless you consider references to Camilla sexual. We have a large number of sexual thoughts each day. Estimates vary, but they are all rather surprisingly large. Rumor has it you…oh never mind, it's best not to go there! Unfortunately, the above example doesn't include the visual aspects of our thoughts. Visualizing something is a way of thinking about something, too. Much of our thinking is visual or accompanied by visualizations, and we can react to those visualizations as we do other thoughts, because they are a form of thought. Some people, such as Dr. Temple Grandin, who has autism, are unable to think abstractly. Dr. Grandin explains that her thoughts are all visualizations. She's done quite well for herself, which attests to the power of visual thoughts. The point is: thoughts are not simply words. Words and language may aid thinking, but we would still have thoughts if we had no language or words. Being able to "think about how we think," which we're doing now, makes us uniquely human. Let's put this remarkable ability to good use.

SOME AUTOMATIC THOUGHTS ARE POWERFUL!

Some automatic thoughts inject themselves into our stream of consciousness, and many seem to follow a theme. The ones with which we're most concerned tend to be evaluative (often self-evaluative) or try to predict the future. Depending on the particular thought, it can either lead to feelings of happiness, contentment and pride, or on the opposite extreme, fear, anxiety, sadness, or hopelessness. Frequently, the same thought continues to "pop up," and it follows us throughout or daily activities. Being aware of our automatic thoughts, and changing them when they work against us or do not promote our sense of well-being, is a key to changing our feelings and behavior. Here's a small sample of some positive and negative automatic thoughts:

POSITIVE AUTOMATIC THOUGHTS
I'm doing a great job
I'm a rock star
I'm proud to have accomplished this
I'm certainly better than average at this
I'm a nice person
I'm making a difference
I handled that well
I've come a long way
I can do it, I'll figure it out
I'm likable and lovable
It will be okay

I'm strong and able to handle what is thrown my way
Things will be okay in the future
I'm going to have fun
Working hard makes me stronger no matter the result
I will not let my perfectionism get in the way of my progress

NEGATIVE AUTOMATIC THOUGHTS
I'm an idiot!
I'm a loser!
I'm so stupid!
I'm not very good at this
I'm unappreciated
I'm embarrassed because…
My efforts aren't appreciated
I screw everything up
One step forward, two steps backward
I know I'll hate it
Things won't get better
I'm going to get in over my head and fall apart
I have too many weaknesses
I'm not very likable or lovable
Everything is a struggle
No one really likes me; they're just using me to get what they want
People suck!
I suck!
I'll never get all this done!
I've failed every time, so I'll fail now
I'm never happy, I'm always sad

THOUGHTS TRIGGER FEELINGS

Thoughts trigger feelings, and our feelings trigger our behavior. Another way of saying this is our thoughts create our emotions and our emotions drive our behavior.

A thought can be compared to a snowball, and a snowball can sometimes lead to events that result in an avalanche of feelings and emotions. Like avalanches, acting on some feelings can sometimes create quite a mess, or at the least not have the outcome we desire. Once avalanches or strong feelings arise, it is hard to stop them. It takes an enormous amount of restraint not to act on some of our feel-ings, sometimes more strength than we have. That kind of extreme restraint, while useful in one way, is very bad for our health. It would be much easier to change the thought (snowball) than the resulting emotion (avalanche) or try to block (restraint) the avalanche from occurring and causing havoc. To add to this catastrophe, we are often also stuck dealing with our reaction to the mess we caused (feeling guilty, remorseful, or otherwise lousy)! The way to change outcomes is to change the original thought.

If Snowballs Were Thoughts

I started an avalanche that hit a small town,
When it hit, it knocked everything down.
It started quite quietly, just a bit of soft snow,
But it led to the start of an avalanche flow.

The damage done was truly not sought,
Just a snowball I tossed, no more than a thought.
But it tumbled and tumbled down the steep slope,
And grew larger and larger, against all my hope.

It surely wasn't planned, this sad end result,
So, is the damage it caused really my fault?
It was just a small thought tossed in the air,
But the damage done is in need of repair.

The point of this story, and I'm sure you agree,
Is to show how powerful even small thoughts can be.
If snowballs are thoughts and avalanches emotion,
It's a new way of thinking, quite a powerful notion!

If you think about it, the concept that thoughts cause feelings that lead to behaviors makes common sense. Certainly, you can get in touch with your feelings, because they are also physiological, but your interpretations of those feelings are thoughts. Looking at our behavior this way was developed by Aaron Beck in the 1960s as a form of therapy. His aim was to change counterproductive (he called it "dysfunctional") thinking, behavior, and our reactions. It is a way of breaking free from patterns that work against us, and ultimately a way of taking more control over our lives. He called his approach "cognitive-behavioral therapy". It is a beautiful approach in that it is easy to understand and highly effective.

Some of Us Can't See the Connection

Many of us have a hard time accepting we have power over our thoughts. We think the snowball jumps into our hands and some supernatural power makes our arm throw the snowball. We just don't think about our thinking, or don't believe we can change the way we think. This is evident in some very common responses:

- That's just the way I am!

- I am who I am, and that's it! (Did we learn part of this from Popeye?)

- That's just my style!

- That's the way I do things!

The truth is you can change how you think (and therefore how you feel and do things). You are constantly changing who you are. The person you were yesterday is a bit different than the person you are today. If you accept the challenge to change some of your thoughts, you can change some of your counterproductive or destructive patterns, and hence, change your life. Because some thinking patterns are harmful in that they lead to overeating, you have three choices:

1. Change your thinking that leads to overeating

2. Use constant restraint (if you even can) to block overeating

3. Continue on the path you are on and accept the results

MOST THOUGHTS ARE AUTOMATIC

Our lives are based on patterns and routines. This is very useful, or we'd be stuck figuring out our daily routine from scratch each morning. Even our biology has rhythms and cycles. We are programmed to repeat things. It is part of the package deal we inherited. Fortunately, we don't have to figure things out from scratch each new day. Once we establish a routine, we like to stick to it unless we make a conscious effort to change it. We often screw things up if there is an unexpected change in our routine. We get up in the morning, sit at the edge of the bed for a minute, convince ourselves we can move ahead, put on our slippers, and usually head to the bathroom to pee. We do this without trying to think about it; the thoughts are automatic. If we get any of the steps out of sequence, we'll have to explain the puddle next to the bed. Unless we purposefully "think about our thinking," thoughts are usually effortless, unending and often follow the same patterns and habits. Your thoughts, however, are unique to you, and the script for your thoughts is different from the rest of us. All your scripts are written by the same author, you—intentionally or more likely, unintentionally. For example, you may think about your day's work schedule every day while you shave. Unless we put effort into it, our thoughts are automatic. If something throws us off our regular routine, it can have a rippling effect and even have serious consequences. If you usually don't take the garbage out with you when you go to work, but decide one day to do so, you may find yourself in the subway or in your car holding a bag of garbage. Most of our thoughts are not purposeful; they are automatic and seem to just pop into our heads. This can be a problem when it comes to food and eating.

RESPONDING TO REAL LIFE-THREATENING SITUATIONS

We have countless automatic thoughts and reactions, and many of them are related to feeling threatened in some way. Before we can appreciate how we react to non-life-threatening situations as if they are life-threatening, we first want to look at how we react to real life-threatening situations. When we sense our life is at stake, we react immediate, with little if any thought. It is as if an alarm button is pushed. Life threatening feelings mobilize our bodies to deal with extremely dangerous situations. This increases our chance of survival. Our body prepares us by generating a "fight, flight, or freeze" (FFF) response. For example, imagine you are on an African safari and venture off the Jeep to take a closer look at a majestic lion. Then, imagine your driver, annoyed that you didn't tip him for yesterday's excursion, slowly drives away, humming, "The lion sleeps tonight". Now it's just you and the lion. The lion, thankful for the home delivery, licks his chops, stares squarely at you, and starts to amble straight toward you. If you have the thought, "I need to get out of here now," that would be

100% accurate, because this is truly a life-threatening situation. The lion, you anticipate, is likely going to eat you if you do not do something, and you "need" to act quickly. After the "need" thought crosses your mind in a flash, your body is then instantly going to turn on the FFF response. It wastes no time; it's a flick of the switch and not the product of careful deliberation.

THE FIGHT, FLIGHT OR FREEZE RESPONSE

The fight, flight or freeze (FFF) response is your body's way to save your life. Your body releases hormones into your bloodstream that immediately give you energy. The primary hormones released are adrenaline (also known as epinephrine), which you probably heard of, and cortisol, which you may or may not have heard something about. For diabetics, cortisol is an important chemical. The adrenaline gives you an immediate and huge surge of energy. It gives you the energy to fight the lion or run like hell. Both adrenaline and cortisol take sugar out of storage from your liver and muscles. This is the fuel you'll need to save your life. Survival is the only important thing on your agenda, and the adrenalin gives you "tunnel vision" enabling you to focus exclusively on your survival. In some cases, we may also "freeze". You see many animals do this to lessen the odds they will be noticed. Because the lion is staring at you and grinning, you know he sees you, so it is less likely you will freeze like the proverbial "deer in the headlights". We, like other animals, can become so frightened that we freeze and lose control of our bodily functions. It really is possible to scare the s*&% out of someone. Please don't put this book down to test this on an unsuspecting neighbor. However, back to our lion; he is already picking out just the right wine to have with you (a South African Chardonnay probably), so you are going to need to fight or take flight. If the lion or any other animal comes after you and bites you, it will first probably bite your arm or leg. In preparation, nature has thoughtfully moved much of your blood away from your arms and legs to the center of your body. In addition, the cortisol that is released along with the adrenaline reduces inflammation from the bite. Together, these two responses increase your odds of survival, although in this case, the bookies strongly favor the lion.

Remember that our ancestors survived by overeating to survive famine (which is usually part of our overeating problem). Well, in addition to those genes having a better chance of survival, so too were those ancient ancestors who had strong FFF responses. They had the competitive edge and passed their genes on to us. Those who had weak FFF responses became main entrees, because they were unable to fight or flee as quickly. Modern humans excel at the FFF response, usually too well for our modern lifestyles. Soldiers, police officers, firefighters and criminals might find this trait extremely useful, but for the majority of us, we seldom encounter life-threatening situations on a daily basis. Although the FFF response better insures survival, it takes its toll on the body. It is similar to the harm caused by racing a car's engine; it is simply not good for a car. Our problem is that the way we think can cause our body to react as if we are in a life-threatening situation when it is not one. It takes a heavy toll on us, and is the root of why we feel stressed and anxious.

NEEDS VS WANTS: FFF IN LESS THAN LIFE-THREATENING SITUATIONS

We generate many life-threatening type thoughts, even when we are not in life- threatening situations. They're a big problem. Most life-threatening thoughts are not responses to true life-threatening situations. Feeling like, "I *must* get out of here," because your boss is driving you too hard might set off your FFF response even if you still have five more hours of work, and even if your boss wouldn't hurt a fly. The FFF response releases adrenaline and unless it is a true emergency, it gives us more energy than we need. We often call this extra energy "nervous energy". We end up with this extra energy because we confuse our "needs" with our "wants". In effect, we trigger our own FFF states by the way we think. We do this because we believe whatever pops into our heads, which, of course, are our own thoughts! In reality, all we *really* "need" are oxygen, water, a small amount of food, and shelter from extreme elements. We don't really "need" a snack, a coffee break, a new job, or the 10 extra minutes more used to reach our destination because of heavy traffic. We might "want" them, but we don't "need" them. However, many of us have the very bad habit of thinking about or talking about some of our "wants" as "needs". More often than not, we do this silently when we talk to ourselves. We may not even be aware of it. When we do this, however, we trigger our FFF response. Yes, part of our brain is listening and waiting for triggers. That's its job. It's very good at it and believes what we tell it. Remember, only those ancestors with the best FFF responses survived to pass their genes. They must have been nervous wrecks!

FFF and Short-Term Thinking

Our brain is programmed to stay in a short-term thinking mode when our FFF response is triggered; it is our default setting and we remain there long after the real or imagined threat has left. The short-term thinking part of our brain, sometimes referred to as the ancient (or primitive) part of our brain, has both a sadly limited vocabulary and bad hearing. It hears and understands the word "need" quite well. In fact, it is so well-programmed to hear and satisfy basic needs that it will often mishear "want" as "need". When our brain hears us use the word "need" when we talk to ourselves or others, it raises our anxiety, and we are compelled to act urgently. Because of its hearing deficit, it hears, "should," "must," "got to," "have to," etc. as "need". Holding an intelligent, rational conversation with this ancient part of our brain is impossible. However yell, "Boo!" and it understands the message very well!

When we are thinking in the short-term mode, which is much of the time, we don't have very good filters for the overwhelming number of automatic thoughts that pop up. For example, if a thought such as, "I *need* to eat this piece of pizza," pops into our head, we actually experience the *need* to eat the pizza, and we experience it the same way we experience the *need* to breathe—yes, as ridiculous as that sounds! In actuality, we don't really *need* the pizza unless we are at the brink of starvation. If you have not started gnawing on the corners of this book, chances are you are not at the brink of starvation. To actually *need* something would imply your life is in immediate danger. Again, when we think in words such as "need to," "have to," or "must," we're going to actually *feel* that we're in a life-threatening situation and act accordingly. Yes, it is strange, but it is also true.

The problem with short-term mode thinking, once it is triggered by hearing "need," is that it is not programmed to encourage us to stop and objectively reevaluate our situation. To stop and evaluate would defeat the purpose of the FFF survival response. You don't stop to reevaluate your situation when a lion is charging at you. Those reflective, analytical ancestors who stopped to contemplate their situations didn't quite make it home. That's the whole darn problem with short-term mode thinking and FFF! We're wired to respond to "need," "must," "require," etc. as if we're in an emergency situation even when it is not an emergency. This leads to problems such as overeating, because we feel we *need* to eat when we don't really need to eat. Remember, eating also relaxes us, temporarily reducing our anxiety. If we are going to lose weight, we want to stop allowing "need" and "food" from existing in the same thought. This is not going to happen unless we make a conscious effort to listen to ourselves and think about our thinking. When "food" and "need" share the same thought, we can catch it and switch to the long-term, rational part of our brain, and remind ourselves that we "want" food, we don't "need" it. We can also trigger our long-term thinking by reminding ourselves of our long-term goals. You turn off the short-term thinking by turning on the long-term thinking…and sticking with it! Don't think you can get away with flicking the switch, leave it on! Let your long-term, rational part of your brain take control of your decision making.

FFF and Tunnel Vision

Getting your long-term thinking part of your brain to take over is "Easier said than done". It will take effort to switch from short-term to long-term thinking on command. You might want to think about your thinking to accomplish this. If you have the ability to learn how to use the buttons on a remote control to change channels (not to be confused with the more complicated task of programming the remote), you have the ability to learn how to switch from short-to long-term thinking on demand (although it might take a bit more practice). You will want to first be aware of one important thing: tunnel vision. Part of the challenge you'll face switching from short-term thinking to long-term thinking is tunnel vision. Tunnel vision is part of the FFF response and vital in life and death situations. The tunnel vision helps us deal only with the emergency at hand by minimizing distractions. Tunnel vision causes us to dismiss other thoughts and sensations so we can focus exclusively on the task at hand, which for us is often eating. We focus on food and consume whatever we can get our hands on, as if we are literally starving. We reveal our mindset when we use common declarations such as, "I'm starving to death!" when asked if we're hungry. Ever catch yourself eating at a pace more appropriate to a pie eating contest at a country fair than dinner at home? Wonder what the heck is happening? Now you know the answer. If we don't consciously intercede between our thoughts and our eating, we'll eat as if our lives depend on it. The body and the mind cannot be separated. *The Greenwich Diet* is as much about feeding our brain wholesome thoughts as much as it is about feeding our body foods that help us lose weight and take better control of our diabetes.

Change "Needs" into "Wants"

Much can be accomplished by using the term "want" instead of "need" when referring to food. It is a simple exchange of words. Sure, this sounds silly, but it works. By flagging the word "need" and replacing it with the word "want" we can avoid unnecessary anxiety and unhealthy behavior. Outside of extreme situations, food is a want, not a need. Get your red flag ready and start waving it each time you think the words "need," "eat," or "food" in the same sentence. Waving the flag not only catches you in time, but helps activate your long-term thinking. Once you are engaged in long-term thinking, stay there. Unless your life is truly at stake, long-term thinking will help you make much better decisions in all types of situations, except, of course, real threatening situations.

Help I'm Trapped!

Be aware that nervous energy can also result in a "freeze" response. The freeze response is the third and frequently neglected member of the FFF team. It's actually sometimes hard to recognize, because it feels more like a silent panic, or like you are paralyzed and *can't* fight or flee. This likely happens because fighting or fleeing is often impractical, and we've been trained to stifle those reactions (running when you see your boss is frowned upon unless he or she is your track coach) or socially unacceptable (fighting is usually unlawful unless it follows "sporting rules"). Instead of fighting or fleeing, when we freeze we feel trapped, immobilized, and nervous. Our brain freezes and everything we do seems to suffer. Our blood sugar is elevated as a result of the hormones released, and our ability to think clearly is impaired. Being highly anxious because of the FFF response is one of the most uncomfortable emotional states we can experience. Because it feels so uncomfortable, we'll do anything to get out of it. Too often, we use our impaired judgment to find a solution to our discomfort: food.

Food, you remember, is very comforting, and seems to be the perfect choice when your judgment is impaired. However, eating helps only for a short while; it is a bit of a set up. To keep the anxiety down, you'll want to continue eating. Sound familiar? Taken to an extreme, however, anxiety can also produce the opposite response and make us sick to our stomach. You'll want to raise your red flag when you feel the "need to eat". When the red flag goes up, consciously switch to your long-term thinking. You can then remind yourself of the importance of your commitment and the progress you've made on your long-term goals. Keep your eye on the horizon.

Exercise for Quick Relief

Because feelings such as anxiety tend to stay around longer than needed, like an engine that takes time to cool, we're often left with a residual supply of "nervous energy". When this energy is used for movement, such as walking or running, you effectively "burn off" the extra adrenalin. This is why exercise is such an effective form of treatment for anxiety. Without burning off the adrenaline, nervous energy feels dreadful.

FFF AND FOOD

Food shuts off the FFF response quickly. Just thinking of your favorite food often relaxes your body. This is because the opposite of the FFF response is relaxation. You can't be anxious and relaxed at the same time; relaxation is the antidote for anxiety. The relaxation and digestion system (which we'll simply refer to as the RD system) is in charge of digestion, relaxing, most of our sexual behavior, and a host of other things. The RD system feels really good when it is turned on, and eating does a great job of turning it on. The RD response feels as good as the FFF response feels bad.

It is natural that when anxious because the FFF response is triggered, you try to turn the terrible feeling off with the RD system. It is a perfect solution…well, at least temporarily. Because we have tunnel vision from the adrenalin, we really can't focus on any long-term consequences or goals. We're in the short-term thinking mode, and that's that. We want immediate relief, know how to get it, and we act on it with lightning speed.

Each of us manages our FFF response differently, and we have ways to turn it off quickly. Many of us turn to food to turn the response off. In fact, *there is no quicker way to turn off the FFF response than eating!* It is also socially acceptable. Hey, we often call our most calming foods "comfort food"! Ever wonder why?

Sometimes our FFF response is so extremely intense it cannot be overwritten by the RD (relaxation and digestion) response. This is our body screaming, "Don't you dare eat; you are in danger!" When this happens you cannot eat. You feel sick to your stomach and sometimes you even vomit. For most people, public speaking is so feared it elicits our FFF response even more than death. Imagine, we would rather face death than speak publicly before an audience. For some of us, it has the same degree of fear that our ancestors had of being eaten alive. Because public speakers are usually not eaten by displeased audiences, you can see that thoughts are as powerful as reality. To avoid problems that result from our FFF response, we want to outsmart our thoughts. We want to think about our thinking and feed our mind.

YUM, THIS IS SO DELICIOUS IT COULD BE ADDICTING!

Remember, in addition to the FFF response, we are programmed to eat copious amounts of food when it is available. We inherited both the feast or famine program as well as the FFF response, a real double whammy. The way nature ensures we feast is by rewarding us with a release of the neurotransmitter called dopamine. Dopamine in our brain makes us feel happy. Lots of dopamine results in euphoria. By eating, we do three things:

1. Turn off the fight-flee-freeze response
2. Turn on the relaxation and digestion response
3. Release the happy neurotransmitter dopamine

EATING IS ADDICTIVE

There is emerging evidence that overeating, like some drugs, can be addictive. For example, methamphetamine (meth, crystal meth, Tina, etc.) releases a tremendous amount of dopamine into the brain, more than any other known substance. Because dopamine feels so fantastic, we are driven to continuously have that feeling. When dopamine drops, the brain seeks an increase to bring it up to the level it just had. It demands we "do" it again. The drive is so strong that it takes priority over all else. Satisfying the brain becomes a way of life, a lifestyle. It is no coincidence that the first two letters of "dopamine" are "do". When addicts say, "There is nothing as good as that first high," they are actually saying that a dopamine expectation level was set upon their first use, and life becomes dedicated to trying to relive that initial high.

Food follows this same path, but obviously on a much diminished scale. Food doesn't raise our dopamine level as high as meth, but it does raise it substantially. When we stop eating, our dopamine levels drop, and we look for a refill of happiness by eating. We can turn a negative emotional state into an extremely positive state simply by grabbing some chips. Scary.

THE SIX HEAVY DOPAMINE HITTERS

The six activities that increase our dopamine and lead to addictive behavior are: eating, drinking, drugging, gambling, shopping, and sex. Of these, food is both readily available and socially acceptable. If you do drugs on the job, have sex on your desk, toast your boss with a shot of tequila at each meeting, meet openly with your bookie, or constantly shop on the Internet, you'll likely be fired. We don't openly take shopping breaks, sex breaks, or drug breaks, but we take food breaks. No one blinks an eye if you tear open a bag of corn chips, a bag of cookies, or partake of the spread laid out for important meetings.

You can always depend on your good buddy, food, to lift your spirits. When under pressure, and with work backing up, a handful of chocolates will increase your dopamine, turn off your FFF response, and relax you with the RD response. When facing an insurmountable task, we often tackle it with food.

We are so used to eating to relieve anxiety that sometimes we go as far as to eat in anticipation of facing bad events or a bad day. We lower our anxiety so often this way that it becomes a way of life, or more accurately, a trap. Eating is as automatic as driving a car, and you don't need a license.

It sometimes seems there is no better way of getting through a period of negative emotions than eating. It is a wonderful short-term solution. In the long run, however, it destroys us with weight gain and diabetes. The short-term solution comes at too great a cost. Unfortunately, most of our brain is dedicated to short-term projects. If we want to keep the long-term consequences in mind, it takes a conscious effort. Our brain will automatically remind us of short-term rewards, but we'll have to remind ourselves of the long-term rewards because they are not automatic…yet. No magic fairy is going to do this for us, and our brain is not going to take over our long-term life management on its own. Our brain is like a credit card; it focuses on short-term needs and wants until we accrue more debt than we can manage. For us who are overweight and have diabetes, the bill collector is at our door, and it is time to develop a long-term plan to pay off our debts. Losing weight and controlling our diabetes will take work, but if we do it the right way, it will not require us to feel deprived, be constantly hungry, or rely on extraordinary willpower.

When we become more aware of our thoughts, which we can do by thinking about our thinking, we usually learn two different things:

1. We generate an untold number of automatic thoughts each day. Some of those thoughts build us up, and others put us down. Those automatic thoughts are like bad habits, and they pop up unintentionally. Through awareness of our thinking, and then practice and repetition, we can change those negative automatic thoughts to positive ones. The magic is that we believe and react to what we tell ourselves. Tell yourself often enough that you're fantastic and you will feel fantastic. Tell yourself you are stupid, and you will feel stupid. Feelings come from our thoughts and positive thoughts lead to feeling good. When we feel good, we rely less upon food to alter our feelings. Prevention is worth a pound of chocolate.

2. The way we think of things and the words we use when we think often put us into a state of heightened alertness. Our body and mind react to demanding and scary words such

as "must," "should," and "need" with the FFF response. This is stressful, bad for our body and, fortunately, avoidable. You can change the way you think and talk. Exchange your use of words such as "must" and "should" with "can," and exchange "need" with "want". Feed your brain a new diet. Changing the way you think and the words you use will result in feeling less stress. When you are less stressed, you're less likely to turn to food to relax you.

To face this weight loss challenge and be successful, we want to even the odds by learning how to increase our pleasure by means other than food. Success does not come through deprivation; it comes from discovering new ways to increase our pleasure. We can lose weight, manage our diabetes, create a new way of living, and be happier. It is a win, win, win, and win situation, but we're going to first want to figure out how to increase our pleasure without long-term negative consequences.

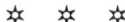

Chapter 12

PLEASURE IS POWERFUL MEDICINE

We do not have to give up pleasure to lose weight! Most people who think about weight loss imagine they have to live a deprived, highly disciplined life, especially in regard to food and exercise. They imagine having to graze almost exclusively on salads and exercise in spite of pain. Self-discipline is fine if you have a good plan; the problem is that most people have a lousy plan—one full of pain, hard work, and constant hunger. Many weight loss plans expect success in the absence of pleasure and moments of satisfaction. They also treat eating as if it is cut off from the rest of our lives, which it is not. A successful plan has to be comfortable and rewarding enough with which to live permanently. We don't want to exchange happiness and satisfaction for a slimmer body. Being thin but miserable is hardly an attractive goal. Living a life full of pleasure, you'll find, is indeed powerful medicine.

FEARING THE LOSS OF PLEASURABLE FOOD

If much of our pleasure isn't going to come from food, then where the heck is it supposed to come from? The answer is deceptively simple. We've created lives for ourselves in which our brains "think" they know exactly what they like and dislike. We sometimes have the mistaken notion that our brain is rational, intelligent, and trustworthy. Sure, parts of our brain are, but some parts still function as it they did millenniums ago. For lack of a better word, we'll call it the "ancient" (or "primitive") part of our brain, as opposed to the more "modern" part of our brain that is more advanced and rational. The ancient part of our brain has more to do with bodily functions, and the modern part of our brain gets us to figure out how to land on mars. The ancient and modern parts of our brain are not always in agreement—and that's why thinking about our thinking is so important. We often make the mistake of forgetting that some parts of our brain that influence our behavior, including eating, are extremely outdated. Our brain is not totally adapted to living in the modern world. You might have assumed your brain "thinks" it knows exactly what it likes and what it dislikes… but no, it doesn't…that would make your life too easy! Our brain makes mistakes, very large mistakes! This is responsible, in great part, for our excess weight. If our brain is so spiffy, why would we be in the situation we're in? The answer is not because we're stupid. Stupidity is not the cause of weight gain.

ARE YOU A VICTIM OF POOR PLEASURE PREDICTIONS?

One extremely common mistake our brain makes is not being able to accurately predict pleasurable upcoming events. Recall this snafu is called "poor pleasure prediction," or simply PPP. It is a mental (cognitive) distortion concerning what we expect. For example, you might have PPP when a friend suggests you go to the park and play Frisbee. You *think* you won't have much fun, but there is a good chance that you will. There is a greater chance that it will be a blast, but your brain *thinks* the plan stinks. So even if you begrudgingly go, your brain likes to prove it is right and will try to convince you a bad time awaits you even after you decide to go. However, more often than not, once you get to the park and find yourself in a new situation, your sense of pleasure changes too. We've all said, "Boy, I'm glad I came," after being dragged tooth and nail to some event or another. Sadly, we repeat PPP next time a similar event occurs, even though we "remember" our forecasts have been wrong in the past.

It is essential that you accept the fact that your brain will tell you to avoid things you are planning (or thinking about planning). Do not be tricked into expecting the worst from your new exercise, your new diet, or your new lifestyle. When you don't want to do something you know will be beneficial to you, just go ahead and do it anyway. The hardest part is just getting to the location or taking the first step. If you know walking is good for you, get outside or go to a park. If you think a recommended meal will leave you feeling deprived, just start cooking. Things begin to change once the first step is taken. "Just show up," is an important philosophy by which to live. Don't "ponder" whether or not you really want to do something good for yourself; just do it. Things will begin to change if you just start "showing up".

DEPRESSION AND PPP

If we are depressed, we probably have a PPP problem. Forcing oneself out into the real world is pivotal in treating depression. One of the fundamental problems with depression is that those of us who are depressed isolate ourselves and PPP all day long. We create living conditions devoid of pleasure, and predict more of the same. Often, depressed people turn to eating, drinking, drugging, gambling, sex, or shopping to increase their pleasure. The remedies are powerful, because in the short-run they work immediately. In the long-run, however, they can destroy lives. Yes, some people destroy themselves in the pursuit of short bursts of happiness. Happiness is that important.

If we're depressed, we sometimes come to the conclusion that, "All I really like to do is eat." Eating, of course, produces short-term pleasure and relaxation, both of which a depressed person strongly desires. Even the negative automatic thoughts sound a bit better when we're eating, and our heavy feelings seem temporarily lighter, because eating can override negative feelings. If we stop eating, the pleasure quickly fades. We're then left feeling overly full and our elevated blood sugar level adds to our negative feelings. But we're not done yet. The worst part comes once we reflect upon our overconsumption. Self-criticism follows: "You fat pig, what the hell did you do that for? You know better!" We call ourselves "losers," feel doomed, and predict we'll end up eating ourselves to death. The name calling alone is self-destructive and we feel terrible both doing it and being the brunt of our own anger and frustration. But you don't have to feel horrible constantly if you don't want to; the remedy is always within your reach: food. Nobody feels totally horrid if there is food around. We can get a respite from our negative feelings by eating more…ah, pleasure once again! We repeat this pattern and spiral downward. Often, we are unaware of the true extent of our nosedive:

Overeat to Feel Good Cycle

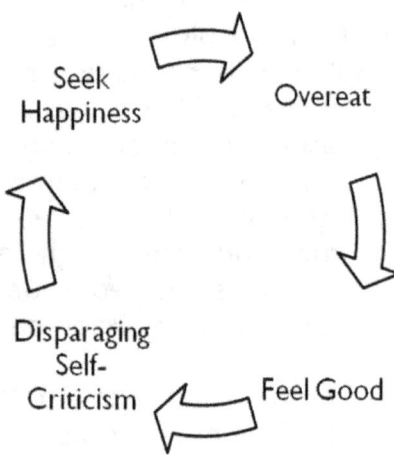

Seek Happiness

Overeat

Feel Good

Disparaging Self-Criticism

The downward spiral is often gradual, and we eat to cope, but we also know it is not working for us. No one has to feel horrible for long if there is food around, but there are better coping strategies than eating. To break this downward spiral, we can attack it from two directions: (1) We can change our thoughts so that we don't feel bad in the first place, and/or (2) We can change our behavior as it relates to this downward spiral.

Here's the downside, the bad news, the thorny challenges we face:

1. Nothing legal can compete with food when it comes to so-cially acceptable short-term pleasure and mood change. Sorry for the bad news.

2. Exercise is not likely to help either. When we feel bad we want pleasure, and we want it now! Exercise is wonderful, benefi-cial, and recommended, but it's not going to help lift your mood immediately. Exercise will help us feel better, but not quickly enough to replace eating.

Here's the upside:

1. There are alternative ways to elevate your mood and have pleasure.

UNDERSTANDING PLEASURE

If we are to be successful, we will want to find alternative sources of pleasure. There are two types of pleasure: mastery and hedonistic pleasure.

Hedonism: The term "hedonism" is often misused, giving it the mystique of being selfish, excessive, naughty, animal-like, or sexy, and some dictionaries say it is, "the relentless pursuit of pleasure". We don't have to be "relentless" about it, but we all desire pleasure; there's nothing wrong with wanting pleasure. Pleasure feels good; it gives us the "oohs" and "aahs" in life. Hedonistic pleasure is a result of dopamine surging though our brain, and it feels physiologically wonderful. Hedonistic pleasure hits quickly and we love it! Examples of hedonistic pleasures are sex, buying a new car, sex, winning at the slot machines, sex, taking some illicit drug, sex, having a glass of wine, sex, or....eating.

Mastery: The other type of pleasure is mastery pleasure. Mastery pleasure doesn't provide dopamine to our brain while we're performing the task. Mastery pleasure requires patience. The dopamine that provides pleasure comes when we finish the task. It is the joy and pleasure that come from an accomplishment. Exercise is a wonderful form of mastery pleasure. While it doesn't bring happiness while we do it, once completed, it provides a sense of achievement. We get our dopamine hit after we complete our exercises. Incidentally, exercise also burns off adrenaline, which makes us feel relaxed. Mastery pleasure, unlike hedonistic pleasure, takes a lot longer, but it is almost always free of long-term negative consequences. Better, it is almost always filled with long-term rewards!

PLEASURABLE SUBSTITUTES FOR EATING

Don't think about "giving up" some of the hedonistic pleasure you get from food. Instead, think about substitutes for that pleasure. When substituting the pleasure obtained from eating, stick to socially acceptable substitutes please. Substituting one hedonistic pleasure for another, something that happens all too frequently, can destroy lives. The unacceptable ones, as a reminder, are drinking alcohol, gambling, illicit drugs, shopping, and sex when taken to an extreme. These substitutes, along with food are the "heavy six" coping mechanisms. Each, however, leads to its own long-term problem; you are already intimately familiar with at least one of the six: food.

The above coping mechanisms are all like short-acting drugs that require frequent doses. The best substitute for food is to seek long-acting, mastery pleasure. Think of it as a time-released dose of pleasure, a sustained dose of pleasure. You'll want to do some self-exploration and ask yourself, "What do I like to do that doesn't involve food and that brings me pleasure?" Engaging in fun and pleasurable activities is vitally important if we want to lessen our reliance upon food for pleasure. Don't get trapped into the, "Nothing is better than food," excuse. We are not looking for pleasures equal to or better than food, that's a set up for failure. We're simply looking for some other source of pleasure. Identifying healthy alternative sources of pleasure is extremely difficult for many people. Some of us are not engaged in many activities and claim we have no other interests.

If you're having a hard time identifying pleasurable activities, think back to what you enjoyed when you were a child. Children are pleasure seekers and do an exceptional job of finding pleasure. That's why most children are very happy and why we often wish we could be a child again. What you enjoyed as a child likely reflects things you could reintroduce into your life. Did you enjoy playing an instrument? Did you like shooting hoops, swimming? Did you like video games? How about board games? Did you like playing with dolls, action figures, or animals? Observe a child running around on the playground and watch how they ignore their discomfort as they go into a full sprint and smile afterwards as if they are outrunning the "bad guy". Children are free of the guilt adults place on themselves for enjoying things. If you are looking for pleasurable activities, start turning the clock back in time, and don't judge things as being "too childish". You can also give some thought to those times when you said, "One day I'd like to..." Perhaps, now is your day.

THINK BIG

If you can't find a few activities that fit into your current lifestyle, stand back and look at the whole of your life. See the big picture. Many adults believe that they "shouldn't" experience pleasure or are ashamed of non-traditional pleasure. This continued denial can become a way of life, a lifestyle. Think of the disgruntled billion-dollar businessman scoffing at the surfer. He thinks, "That burned out surfer dude should be working, the lazy...." and then he proceeds to dream of his steak dinner and martini fiesta that will get him through the rest of his dreaded work day. The surfer might have little money, but receives mastery pleasure from his activity. There are no long-term negative consequences from the surfing (if he uses sunscreen and avoids sharks). Perhaps one could argue that the surfer could be making a better living if he exchanged the wetsuit for a Brooks Brothers suit, and indeed he probably could make more money. But would he be happy? Bottom line is that it's worth more than a billion dollars if an individual knows how to engage in an activity that raises their dopamine levels with no negative long-term consequences. That's real wealth! Your mission is to find your pleasures in life.

If we engage in fun activities, our dopamine level will rise. We'll feel good as well as decrease the odds that we will seek out food to elevate our mood. Don't set yourself up for failure by expecting your activities to raise your dopamine level to where it was when you were overeating. On a scale of 1 to 10, eating scores a solid 10. Don't expect your substitute activities to do the same. You might place your satisfaction level at a 5 or 6, which is far below a 10. But a 5 or a 6 is neutral, and an okay place to be. You won't feel elated, but at least you'll feel okay. Better, you will not have to endure those self-disparaging thoughts, or those lows that lead you to overeat. If one source of pleasure is not working for you, such as eating, it makes sense to explore alternative means of obtaining and experiencing pleasure. You might have to experiment a bit, and while you do, remember the PPP. Don't predict you won't like the new activity. Just show up. An old Buddhist proverb sums it up nicely: "Remember, if you are facing the right direction, all you have to do is keep walking."

CHANGING HOW YOU THINK TO BETTER CONTROL BLOOD SUGAR AND LOSE WEIGHT

You now know that what we think leads to our feelings and behaviors. Fortunately, we have the ability to change how we think. If we change our thinking, our feelings as well as our behavior will change accordingly. Yes, we can better control our blood sugar level and lose weight by simply changing some of our thought patterns. *The Greenwich Diet* includes consuming an abundance of positive thoughts.

Trying to understand all your unique thought patterns and how they affect you is a gargantuan task, so we'll stick to the three biggest types of thoughts that affect your ability to control your blood sugar and weight. Modifying these alone is enough to help you. They are:

- Understanding your motivators
- Finding new pleasures
- Changing your thinking

HOW TO GET AND STAY MOTIVATED

Many of us want to lose weight and better control our blood sugar levels, but feel we lack the motivation to pull it off. Sound familiar? Wanting something is different from having the motivation to acquire it. Sure, we might want more income, but we may lack motivation to get a second job. We've heard the lectures about the dangers of "obesity" and diabetes, so we don't require any more convincing that we "should" lose weight. In fact, we're all tired of hearing the standard lecture. Even Ear Nose and Throat doctors find a way to work in the obesity lecture, which admittedly requires some creativity on their part. Our big problem is not our lack of desire to lose weight; our problem is we just can't motivate ourselves to do it. Desire and motivation are very different. Some of our healthcare providers try to motivate us by scaring us, and yes, they mean well. So perhaps we want to be somewhat more tolerant (if we can bear it without our blood pressure soaring). Every once in a while a "scare job" works to get someone to seek treatment, so it is unfair to say it is always bad. In the long run, however, we can all testify that fear hasn't proven to be very effective—at least for us, and at least in the long run. It might get you to start a diet, but not stick to it. So how are we supposed to get motivated? Where do we find motivation? Is it hiding somewhere? Does it come in pill form? Can we order it over the Internet?

USE POSITIVE MOTIVATORS

Since negative motivators don't work, let's rely upon the positive ones! Actually, positive motivators work very well. The proof is in the commercials for weight loss products. They don't scare you by showing bodily damage or someone having a heart attack. Heck no, they show you a positive image of a beautifully shaped, very sexy, thin body! Hubba, hubba, hubba, that's one mighty fine carrot! Hey, if losing weight will enhance your sex appeal or sex life, it is one powerful motivator! Go for it…seriously!

Positive images in your head are great motivators. Psychologists and other mental health professionals have been using this positive approach for years because it works. A positive approach works for individuals, teams, raising kids, and running businesses. If you want to change your behavior, think of the rewards that will result because of the change in your behavior. If people are asked for the positive rewards of weight loss, they usually come up with two or three examples. Not bad. But put them in a room with a paper and pencil and tell them you'll be back in a half hour and they'll produce a much longer list. If asked, they'll admit that most of the benefits didn't occur to them until they sat back and thought about it. As corny as it sounds, sit back, let your imagination run wild, and let it rip. Create your own list!

THE REWARDS OF WEIGHT LOSS

Are you having a problem identifying the rewards that come with weight loss even after giving it a fair shot? This is part of our problem; we're not accustomed to thinking of ourselves as thinner, at least not in detail. In addition to personal goals that apply only to you, there are rewards that are common to most of us. The problem is negative thoughts often shatter before a positive motivating image can take hold. Once you come up with a positive image, hold onto it! The thought can be slippery, so grasp it tightly when it comes to mind. Think of yourself as feeling lean, strong, attractive, and sexy. When you begin to think in this positive manner, an automatic thought often pops up for some of us. It goes something like, "Who are you kidding? You'll never be like that! You're being ridiculous!" Your positive image vaporizes in an instant and you feel defeated. Rather than accept that automatic put down (and a quite negative one at that!) you want to talk back to your thought. Tell your brain that it is making a mistake, and that you refuse to accept the putdown. If it helps, label the negative thought "resistance" or think of it as your fat trying to protect itself. Tell yourself that you refuse to allow this negative thought to rob you of happiness. Do not accept the negative thought by explaining it away, such as, "That's just me." Get it into your brain that if you think negatively, you'll feel negatively, and behave negatively. When a negative thought emerges, remind your brain that, "Positive thoughts lead to motivation, and negative thoughts are a waste of time and harmful to me."

"Talking to your brain" sounds foolish to many of us. We think that our brain has total control over us and it does the talking, not the listening. The fact is that humans are unique in that they can reflect upon their thinking and change the way they think. It is not suggested you think "positively" like Al Franken's Saturday Night Live character, Stewart Smalley. If you do, please record it so the rest of us can enjoy it!

The idea of "thinking about thinking" is one thing, but when people are told they can talk to their brain, they usually roll their eyes and try to change the subject. Talking to your brain sounds foolish enough, but to suggest that your brain will actually listen to you and believe you seems to enter the realm of ridiculous. As absurd as it sounds, if you are relaxed enough, your brain will believe what it is told. This is why and how hypnosis works. If people can be convinced to strut on stage like a Rhode Island Red, and scratch the floor with their feet like a hungry hen, and do so in front of a live, laughing audience, certainly the mind is open to a few positive rational suggestions! Our minds are more open when are bodies are relaxed. You'll notice that the first thing a hypnotist does is help the person relax: "You are becoming sleepy…" Sending positive messages to yourself when you are relaxed is potent. If your brain believes you when you put yourself down, why wouldn't it believe you when you build yourself up? Conversely, trying to instill ideas in the middle of an anxiety attack is next to impossible. The best you can do is talk your way through it—actually a pretty good strategy (in addition to relaxing which will be discussed shortly).

Be reasonable with your positive images and motivators. Aiming to be the wealthiest person in the world or the first in your family to appear on the cover of *Vogue* is thumbing your nose at reality. If your motivator is off the wall, your brain will constantly reject it as totally out of the question (hopefully!). Your brain will know that no matter how hard you work, it is simply just not going to happen. Reality will have the last word. Keep your goal within the realm of reality—ambitious yes, outside of reality, no.

What often excites people the most is fitting into smaller size clothes, being the thinnest person in your walking group, running a distance you were only able to do many years ago, or hitting a milestone in body weight loss. These are the achievements that get people jumping up and down in happiness. Decreasing your HbA1c (a test to determine the average amount of sugar in your blood over a 3-month period) is nice, but most of us don't find it a cause for raucous celebration.

Once you have the positive image and tell your brain you can do it, you want to spend time thinking about the rewards that come from losing weight and controlling hunger. It is not a one-shot deal. It requires repetition, lots of repetition. If you are having a hard time identifying rewards, this might help:

- Shopping for smaller size clothes
- Looking better
- Having your doctor smiling at you when he or she sees your progress
- Having a person look at you lustfully
- Going anywhere you want unimpeded
- Being "perceived" as more intelligent
- Playing sports better
- Having more energy
- Going out to dinner with confidence
- Having friends and family looking at you with admiration
- Being the picture of health in your later years
- Being a weight loss, diabetes control expert
- Being a good role model achieving goals

Once you identify your motivators, it is very important to remind yourself of them daily. Doing this implants them in your brain. Repetition is a key to success. Hey, it is only fair; we took away the negative thoughts that were automatic, so we want to replace them with automatic positive thoughts. This requires repetition. Also, the more specific your motivators are, the more powerful they are. If you want to keep your motivators private, write them down and hide them in your wallet. Be sure to take your list out three times a day and read through each one. It sounds corny, but it is brain training. Would you rather be corny or fat? The more you look at and think about your motivators, the quicker you will change. Soon, you will begin to automatically think positively about the future and feel great.

WHEN TO SEEK PROFESSIONAL HELP

If anxiety or depression has invaded your thought processes, finding a motivator can be very difficult work. If you can't identify good motivators, you may want to first attend to your anxiety or depression. Seek professional help. Techniques such as motivational interviewing and cognitive behavioral therapy can help you break through the barriers.

One of the great benefits of therapy is that it affords us an opportunity to be totally open. Because therapy is confidential, you have the opportunity to discuss things that may be socially unacceptable, politically incorrect, or highly embarrassing.

DON'T FALL FOR THIS MEAN TRICK!

Let's let Joan give an example of the biggest trick our mind can play:

It is Monday morning, and Joan has been working on losing 25 pounds. She feels as committed as ever and has her usual breakfast of a whole wheat English muffin, egg, and slice of low-fat cheese. She prepares herself for work, stuffs a low-carb/low-calorie snack bar in her purse, jumps on her Harley and heads for work. She's tempted to have one of the doughnuts available at the coffee machine, and is once again proud of herself for passing them up. She takes an early lunch, and heads out with friends to a local restaurant. The smells get to her. Hearing the others order burgers and fries is driving her crazy, but she orders a salad and bowl of soup. She also grabs a roll from the basket. Once finished dining, she feels great again for her achievement. She reminds herself that "Rome wasn't built in a day," and she just added another brick. She eats her snack bar in the afternoon, arrives home and heats up one of the frozen SML carb meals she prepared the prior week. She's acing it. "This is really working," she says to herself. After dinner, she relaxes with her husband in front of the TV after attending to family demands. While settling in, her husband leaves the room for a few minutes and returns from his excursion to the kitchen with a slice of homemade cake his mother brought over earlier. Just seeing that delectable treat causes Joan's dopamine level to rise a little, and her brain starts telling her that she wants some. She is in a hard spot once again. Although one part of her brain (the ancient part) tells her to eat a slice, another part of her brain (the modern part) reminds her that having a slice will undermine her long-term goal of shedding 25 pounds. She is torn. Unfortunately, one part of the brain could care less about her long-term goal; nature has programmed it to eat while she has the opportunity. It is growling, "Feed me, feed me now!" The more rational part of her brain reminds her that her long-term goal is important; she *really* wants to lose weight. The problem is, in actuality, she *really* wants to satisfy *both* parts of her brain! The conflict continues, both parts being rather relentless. Then, it hits her; she has a solution: She decides to eat just a little piece of the tasty food, just a bite. "A fair compromise," she says to herself. Wow, it tastes wonderful and she experiences enormous pleasure. Instantly, she starts to relax, which was the whole point of chilling out in front of the TV in the first place. Then the second wave hits—guilt. Eating the cake is working against her long-term goal, and she'll never lose the 25 pounds this way! She feels weak and terrible about herself. She knows she stepped in it. Then she sees a way out. She thinks, "I'll allow myself this now, and I'll be better tomorrow." Voila, she rids herself of the guilt and no negative emotion is left. Instead, she feels great, is guilt-free, and experiences pleasure without remorse. Her brain loves this, she can eat what she wants; she is free! Since she is free to eat, and the food is readily available, her brain tells her to, "Eat while you can, go for it!" Her blood sugar level spikes, and once her binge eating starts, it continues in high gear. If there are moments of guilt, she reminds herself, "Tomorrow is going to be tough, I know, but I'll make up for it. I promise I'll only eat green vegetables." The big problem is she believes it...every darn time! It might take Joan a few tries, but with the help of her food diary she will eventually be able to break this common but destructive pattern. If she is willing to learn from her mistakes by changing her thinking patterns, she'll be able to achieve her long-term goals. Joan is much like many of us.

Joan did a "cleansing process". We love cleansing processes; they wash away dirt, grime, etc. As in the physical world, we also do mental cleansing, as Joan did, but in Joan's case it is to rid herself of her guilt. Joan washed away her guilt by agreeing to make up for her overeating tomorrow. What Joan did is a common trick, a common way to deal with guilt related to overeating. We do this by making promises to "pay up" in the future. We especially like Monday mornings. Mondays signify a new beginning. If we do well with our diet in the beginning of the week, but binge on Wednesday, it's much easier on Thursday through Sunday to give into short-term goals. After all, we'll get a new start next week.

So, what do we do when we find ourselves in Joan's situation? First, we recognize it for what it is...a trap. You want to tell yourself something like, "This trick has defeated me for decades, and it stops now!" or "Part of my brain, the old ancient caveman part, is making a terrible mistake, a big mistake, and I won't allow it." But most important, remind yourself of what you want, both long-term and short-term. Recognize and acknowledge your intense craving for what it is. Saying, "I want to binge badly, but I also want to lose weight, control my diabetes and be happier," is a powerful reminder. You can also distract yourself by engaging in another activity. It is hard to change your thoughts if you are standing over the cake or even being in the same room with it. If you change your location, your mind may follow.

SCALES: THE GREAT DERAILERS

Scales derail more people trying to lose weight than anything else. If you step on a scale and the number goes up, you know some pretty harsh words will follow. After you stop cursing, you might have thoughts similar to, "This simply isn't working!" or "I'll never lose weight. I did everything right and this is what happens?" If scales are a good measure of body fat, those thoughts would be accurate, but scales are not accurate.

The scale is an outdated measure of your weight loss progress. Scales are so old, they outdate most modern religions. Balance scales have been around for thousands of years. Scales were first used to weigh goods for trade—that is until someone had the bright idea of inventing a spring scale in the mid 1800s. Since then, they've been weighing everything they can get their hands on, but they're much more useful for weighing potatoes than people. Even the bioelectrical impedance analysis (BIA) scales mentioned earlier, primarily the less expensive ones, aren't always any more accurate than regular scales.

Much more accurate measures of your body fat exist, but they are too expensive for home use. Weight loss specialists sometimes have them in their offices. There are underwater weighing tanks, DEXA scans (the gold standard), and MRI analysis. However, for many of us, the notches on our belts, the way our clothes fit, and how we are able to move, are all more accurate measures of weight loss. They also don't require a medical office visit.

You might still be tempted to use the old-fashion scale, especially if you have one at home. Your doctor might also insist on weighing you. You are highly encouraged to take the reading with a "grain of salt," or better a "pound of salt". Your scale is going to be more accurate if you weigh yourself once each week, or better yet once each month, or even once every three months. Yes, we're working hard every day on our weight loss and we'd like to see progress every day, but the last thing you want is discouragement. Some of us hard-headed individuals still insist on stepping on the scale every couple of days. If you chart your "progress" for a few months, you'll find that it ends up lower over time, but there are numerous up and down spikes along the way.

We can do a great job finding things that motivate us and even finding alternatives for some of the pleasure we derived from food, but at the end of the day we're left with our feelings. If our feelings are negative, such as sadness or anxiety, and if food helped us deal with those emotions day in and day out, we want help that is more immediate than the rewards and pleasure derived from long-term goals. Fortunately, there are ways to deal with uncomfortable feelings each and every day leading up to realizing our goals. In fact, they provide the stability we need to achieve our goals.

✳   ✳   ✳

Chapter 13

STRESS BE GONE!

Emotions, which we'll also call feelings, are how we measure the quality of our day, our week, and even our lives. For the most part, our feelings are a result of our thoughts. How we think about things determines our feelings. Fortunately, if we are willing to make the effort to change our thoughts, we can change our feelings. When we change how we feel, we change how we behave—including eating behavior.

FEELINGS ARE IN OUR MINDS AND BODY

Love, hate, happiness, fear, and all other emotions are accompanied by physical changes in our body. Hormones, blood flow, muscle tension, heart rate, etc. are all affected by our emotions. How we feel, therefore, is both in our minds and our bodies. Actually, it is not like our body and mind are two different things. Our mind is our brain, and our brain is part of our body. In fact, our thoughts are measurable biochemical and bioelectrical brain activity.

EMOTIONS AND DIABETES

Much of what we know about the relationship between our emotions and diabetes comes from the research and writings of Richard S. Surwit, PhD from the Duke University Medical Center in Durham, NC. He found that diabetes can directly affect our emotions and our emotions can directly affect our diabetes. For example, both anxiety and depression cause changes in our body chemistry, and those changes can directly affect our blood sugar levels. The relationship between our body and emotions works two ways: (1) our emotions affect our physical body, and (2) our physical body affects our emotions. They influence each other in a way that is actually more like they are engaged in a constant dialogue—thoughts provoke feelings that provoke thoughts that provoke feelings, etc. Although the mind-body connection is interesting, it can be very annoying when it comes to trying to figure out the cause of uncomfortable or negative feelings. When the day comes either your brain or body doesn't affect the other, you've either transcended this realm of physical existence or you've kicked the bucket.

PHYSICAL (PHYSIOLOGICAL) CAUSES OF NEGATIVE FEELINGS

None of us are exempt from experiencing negative feelings. Understanding how to deal with them is an important part of successful weight loss, simply because our feelings are often involved in overeating. The term "comfort food" says it all. However, in some cases, negative emotions have nothing to do with the way we think. Instead, they come from something that is happening to our body that is not a result of thoughts. For example, a medical condition or medication can cause physical changes in our body, and we can experience those changes as feelings. If a medication causes us to feel edgy or short-tempered, for example, we're going to end up trying to interpret or label those sensations; we're going to try to figure out where they are coming from—not always an easy job. As an example, your short temper and desire to throw this book at your spouse might be due to the side effect of a medication rather than his or her bad habit of hogging the remote. However, regardless of the cause of our emotions (medication, thoughts, medical condition), they can affect our blood sugar levels. If you are experiencing emotional problems, that is to say an unusual amount of negative feelings:

1. Rule out an underlying medical condition as the cause or contributing factor to negative emotions.

2. Determine if your feelings are a side effect of a medication or an interaction between medications.

3. Stabilize your blood sugar levels.

ANXIETY INCREASES BLOOD SUGAR

If you are anxious or angry, your body releases hormones such as cortisol and epinephrine. This is part of the FFF (fight, flight, or freeze) response which pulls sugar out of storage and moves it into your blood stream so you have the energy needed to protect yourself or run like hell. If sugar is released into your blood stream, your blood sugar level is obviously going to increase. This holds true for all people, not only those of us with diabetes. In fact, the mere anticipation of being in a stressful situation can cause a release of these stress-related hormones. This kind of reminds us of FDR's famous saying: "The only thing we have to fear is fear itself," but you get the point! It even appears that stress or anxiety may be involved in the onset of diabetes for those predisposed to the illness, although other factors besides stress might also be involved. The good news is that you can improve your blood sugar level by finding ways—or learning ways—to relax. Stress, for a diabetic, is like eating a piece of chocolate cake but without the pleasure.

HIGH AND LOW BLOOD SUGAR LEVELS AFFECT EMOTIONS

It appears depression makes our bodies more resistant to insulin, and this can result in high blood sugar levels. If our blood sugar levels are high (hyperglycemia), we will often exhibit depressive symptoms such as fatigue and feelings of hopelessness. It appears high blood sugar levels diminish serotonin, a condition related to depression. A low serotonin level is experienced as unhappiness. A normal serotonin level helps you feel "okay" or "normal". Fortunately, anxiety as well as our blood glucose levels can be reduced through relaxation exercises. But the relationship between high blood sugar levels and depression appears to work both ways: depression affects our blood sugar level, and a high blood sugar level can result in symptoms of depression. It's a real kick in the pants.

On the other hand, if our sugar is low, (hypoglycemia) we often appear to be drunk. The brain runs primarily on sugar, and when our sugar level is low, our brain is not running at full capacity. This can result in irritability, stubbornness, or grumpiness. To the outside observer, our hypoglycemia often makes us appear we're a "stubborn drunk". Unfortunately, when we're hypoglycemic, our brain is often not working well enough for us to even recognize our own impaired state. Others close to us, however, can often recognize the change. Because many people are reticent to be direct and call us out on our orneriness, be attuned to hints.

SLEEPLESSNESS AFFECTS EMOTIONS

Sleeplessness can also adversely affect our emotions. If we're sleep deprived, our emotions can suffer the brunt of it. In fact, some research suggests that sleep deprivation can lead to an elevated blood sugar level even in non-diabetic individuals. This is a double-whammy: not only are you stuck dealing with negative emotions that result from a lack of sleep, but you also end up with hypergly-cemia to boot! This is why a sleep study is important for many of us trying to control our diabetes and lose weight. If we cannot breathe well due to excess body fat impeding our oxygen intake when we sleep (called obstructive sleep apnea), we become sleep deprived. Also, if we have a high blood sugar level, we often become sleepy and close our eyes and nod out, but we do not sleep "well". Although we appear to be soundly asleep, our bodies are working to clear the excess blood sugar rather than resting. Our sleep, consequently, is not as refreshing as we would like. This is not unlike the person who drinks too much alcohol and "passes out". The body shuts down, the person appears to be sleeping, but his or her body is actually devot-ing its energies to breaking down the alcohol. When a person rises from this unconscious state, either due to excess alcohol or sugar, they are typically groggy and have little energy due to lack of restful sleep. Here's a repeat of some of the symptoms of sleep apnea men-tioned earlier:

- Excessive daytime sleepiness or tiredness
- Not feeling refreshed in the morning
- Gasping or choking at night
- Snoring
- Problems with concentration and memory
- Personality or attitude changes
- Morning or nighttime headaches
- Sour taste or heartburn at night
- Swelling of the legs
- Sweating and/or chest pain at night
- Frequent nighttime urination
- Frequently waking up at night, or frequently tossing or turning

FEELINGS LEAD TO ACTIONS (BEHAVIORS)

We act on our feelings. Sure, our brain helps us plan a course of action, and even throws in some "dos, don'ts and shoulds," but the desire to take some form of action stems from our feelings. It doesn't matter what we accomplished during the day, how many times we screwed up, how much money we earned, or our success at shoplifting. It is how we interpret those events that determine our feelings. Interpretations are a type of thought. As a morbid example, we've all been puzzled when we learn of someone who appears to have everything commits suicide. At the end of their day, they didn't *feel* like living; they didn't *feel* life was worth continuing even in spite of having things we *think* "should" have brought them happiness and satisfaction. Perhaps they *felt* unsuccessful, *felt* afraid of the future, *felt* they were failures in some way, or even *felt* angry and took their life to hurt others. Regardless of all the possible reasons, their action stemmed from their feelings. If they felt differently, they would have acted differently. Although we are all different, we are all the same in that we act on our feelings, and those feelings are a result of our thoughts. In one sense, it doesn't matter if those thoughts are based in reality, are distortions of reality, or even hallucinations; they are all powerful. Yes, we're back to that reoccurring theme: our thoughts lead to feelings and our feelings lead to our behavior. Our thoughts might be rather unrelated to reality at times, but the resulting feelings are always real, very real. It is never the case that we "shouldn't" have certain feelings. It would be more accurate for us to say we "shouldn't" have the thoughts that lead to those feelings. Actually, it is fairer to say we don't "want" those thoughts, rather than being so judgmental and casually tossing "shouldn'ts" around. Yes, you're right, in many situations we can tell ourselves not to act on our feelings, or not to trust them, but that is part of the constant dialogue that occurs between our brain and our emotions.

YOU FEEL WHAT YOU THINK

Feelings are a result of our beliefs and our thinking. If the morbid example above doesn't convince you, consider those individuals who face terrible living situations and insurmountable obstacles yet still beam from ear to ear because they "feel good". We say their "heads" are in a different place (such as in the clouds). They obviously think differently than many of us do, often influenced by their beliefs, and their apparent happiness is bewildering to more than a few of us. Negative thinking sometimes leads us to assume their happiness is due to their "ignorance". Sounds like jealousy, doesn't it? Hah, jealousy is an emotion too, and yes, it comes from a thought, a judgment—a good example of how a distorted belief (a thought) can lead to a particular feeling. How we feel usually comes down to our beliefs, rules we live by, intellectual interpretations, particular styles of thinking (blind spots and filters included), expectations, frames of reference, and ideas—all of which we call "thoughts". Understanding this and learning how to use our thoughts to change our feelings, and ultimately our behavior, can change our lives. In our case, it can help us lose weight and control our diabetes.

CHANGING FEELINGS

Feelings can be changed. More often than not, and if the cause of negative feelings isn't due to such things as an illness or medication, feelings have to be traced back to their cause. The cause is a thought or an interpretation (which is still a thought) of things happening to you. Frequently, the more difficult feeling-thought combos are related to things happening to you that seem to be out of your control. Lack of control is very disconcerting.

Feelings, once they occur, are difficult to change while they are happening. It's much easier to prevent them from happening in the first place. This can be done by changing the thinking that leads to the emotional reaction. Feelings are very strong signals to the brain, and negative feelings are particularly strong signals. Negative feelings are resistant to change, and are "sticky"—they like to hang around well after the event has passed. We sometimes think of these sticky feelings as "moods," emotional states that last far too long. We can usually recognize a negative feeling, but often have great difficulty identifying what thoughts generated the negative feeling. When tracing your feelings back to your thoughts, don't be discouraged if you get off to a slow start or become a bit bewildered; that's part of the process. With some effort, you will become more aware of your feelings and the thoughts that accompany or generate them. In doing so, you'll trace your feelings back to their origin. Remember, thoughts can be ideas, judgments, interpretations, beliefs, or images. We want to be especially aware of the feelings that lead to our overeating, or how we use eating to quickly change our uncomfortable feelings. If you can trace the feelings back to your thoughts, you can take better control of your eating. You might want to first focus on the emotions that sabotage your efforts to lose weight and control your blood sugar, but that's an individual choice.

STEPS TO CHANGING YOUR FEELINGS

You'll notice that changing the way you feel and behave all involve increasing your awareness of how you feel and what you think. It is a gradual process and you might find yourself jumping around a bit from one "step" to another; don't worry about it. Here's how the process works:

1. Is There Really a Problem?

Many of us think of our feelings as "the problem". But our feelings are like a gauge telling us whether or not there's something wrong with our engine. Of course, if there's a problem, the problem is not our gauge, but instead, what the gauge measures. If we're feeling okay, we don't have a problem, and the gauge reading is normal. If we are not feeling okay, however, our gauge (feeling) tells us we have a problem, and it might be a small or a large one. Our gauge will constantly remind us that something is wrong until we resolve the problem. Unfortunately, some of us ignore the warning for a long time, sometimes a lifetime, and some of us even turn to drugs or alcohol as ways to ignore the warnings. Many of us find some relief from our emotional distress by producing the good feelings we rely upon from eating. In a way, we're self-medicating, but the side effects are diabetes and extra weight. Eating seems to help in the short term, but adds to our problems in the long run. Could it be we're a bit too accustomed to short-term solutions to our problems? Hmmm…

The first step toward the solution to any problem is recognizing there is indeed a problem. If there is no solution to a problem, it is not really a problem. If there is no possible solution, it is better to think of it as a "condition" to which you want to adapt. On the other extreme, and while this seems obvious to most, there are a few of us who accept our negative feelings as if they are simply a condition—we tell ourselves it is, "Just the way things are." Or better yet, "Just the way I am." Although we may not like the way we feel, some of us decide to accept and live with our negative feelings rather than face the fact that we have a problem. Here's one reason why: once we label our negative feelings as a problem, we start expecting ourselves to find a solution—and the pressure is on. Some of us are so frightened by the possibility that we aren't up to the challenge of solving our problem, we find it more comfortable to deny we have one in the first place. We are pretty sharp when it comes to recognizing this quality in other people, but rather bleary-eyed when it comes to recognizing it in ourselves. Unhappiness, some of us believe, is simply part of the "human condition". Some of us can back up our belief by quoting 19th-century European philosophers. No doubt a few of us can even spell their names correctly! Brooding philosophers aside, we do not have to live a life dominated by negative emotions. If we feel lousy, we have a problem, and where there's a problem, there's a solution, a way out. Don't think of your problem as a condition.

2.   What's the Problem?

Once you acknowledge that your negative feelings are a problem for you, the next step is to stand back and take a look at your life. You want to identify things in your life that are troubling to you. They can be health related, economic, relationship problems, living conditions, or an illness. "Talking it out," with someone helps immensely, but talking with a professional is even better. Although a bit harder, talking it out with a non-opinionated friend or doing this on your own is possible. Telling your friend they can ask questions, but not make judgments or offer advice, is a good way to start. Be prepared to "correct" them if they break your rules. If they slip up (which one can safely bet they will), stick your fingers in your ears and sing *Yankee Doodle Dandy*. This will usually get your point across. Simultaneously crossing your eyes adds a bit of levity, but can draw unwanted attention if done in public. Worse, you may be asked by strangers to provide entertainment at children's birthday parties.

3.   Lay Out Your Problems

If you have only one problem, or one major problem, consider yourself lucky. Most of us have a number of problems, and we're going to want to sort through them and finally put them in some sort of order. Some of the problems on our list might disappear if we address a larger problem. Once you lay them out in an order that makes sense to you, use your common sense to pick out a problem to work on. Some of us are ready to deal with the biggest problem and some of us do better starting on more modest ones. It's your choice. Remember that success breeds success, and solving one problem often gives you the motivation and practice to solve larger ones. Don't allow yourself to set yourself up for failure. Nothing will stifle your efforts more than failure, so choose something you know you can accomplish.

4.   Become More Aware

Admittedly, this can be hard. Once again having someone to talk to helps. The next best thing to another person is a piece of paper upon which to write your thoughts. This step requires you to become aware of your thoughts, and specifically, your thoughts having to do with the problem. Remember, you are thinking about your thinking, the causes of your feelings. Also remember that feelings can be sticky, like a residue of something that's been "on your mind". Identify all of your thoughts about the problem. It is most useful to become aware of all your automatic thoughts and the constant chatter going through your head. Listen to your thoughts as if you are wire tapping your boss's phone. You'll find your emotions are in line with your head-chatter. Ask yourself the following questions:

- What things in your environment trigger your negative feelings?
- What thoughts seem to pull up other thoughts?
- What are your beliefs and values?
- What are your expectations of yourself and the rules you follow?
- What are your negative self-judgments?
- What do you expect from others?

- When do you start moralizing by thinking in "shoulds and shouldn'ts?"

You may also become aware that some of your automatic thoughts follow a pattern, a sort of "style" of thinking. There are many patterns, and here are some of the more common ones:

- PPP (Poor Pleasure Predicting): This is so common it is worth repeating. It is not being able to accurately predict a pleasurable outcome when planning (or thinking about planning) on doing something, e.g. "I'm not going to like people in my exercise group!"

- Catastrophic Thinking: This is like the above on steroids! It is expecting no good and even harm to come from just about everything you do, e.g., "Everything I do gets screwed up!" It is like always expecting the next shoe to drop.

- Mind Reading: You know this one! We know others who do this, but often fail to see this pattern in ourselves. We "think" our non-verbal cues make things clear, or that any sensitive person, or anyone who really cares about us "should" be able to read us. You have your own examples for this one!

- Moralizing: This is the tendency to base decisions too much on "shoulds," as if there are very limited acceptable or rote ways of doing things, e.g., "My spouse 'should' know not to eat those goodies in front of me! I 'shouldn't' have to ask!" Living in a world of "shoulds" limits your thinking and options, because it limits possible solutions. Worse, we spend our days judging and criticizing. It is not a comfortable way to live (and we annoy the heck out of others).

- Overly Generalizing: Applying what you've learned too broadly, e.g. after finding one condescending doctor in a practice, coming to the conclusion, "They're all arrogant in that office!"

- Projecting Negative Motivations: Assuming that others are less than honorably motivated, e.g., "The authors of this book are just out to make a buck!" or, "She doesn't really like my tie, she said that because she is sucking up!"

- All or Nothing Thinking: This method of trying to control things in life doesn't work well. Thinking, "I would rather not have any pizza at all rather than have to settle for one slice," is just one example.

- Rationalizing: Rationalizing is excuse-making that pretends to use sound logic to sell the idea. Some rationalizations can sound pretty darn good; that's why they're so popular! More than a few of us are so skilled at rationalizing, we help our friends make them up! You may be fully aware you are rationalizing, only somewhat aware that your logic is a bit off, or worse, you may be pulling the wool over your own eyes. "If I don't eat the large slice of cake she hands me, she might think I don't trust her cooking," is an example. If you look for excuses to overeat, there is a good chance you are rationalizing. "We better stop and eat now; there might not be a decent restaurant for many miles!" is a handy traveler's rationalization. "I'll wait until spring to start exercising. This way I can do it in the park where the air is fresher," is another example of rationalizing.

- Devaluing: Devaluing is putting things down you want but can't have. More often than not, it is not that you "can't" have your goal, it has more to do with self-doubting your ability to achieve your goal. Devaluing is an attempt to keep balance and appease your desires. Hey, you have to live with yourself! If you want to lose weight, for example, but believe you can't lose weight, you might start minimizing the rewards of weight loss by convincing yourself that your life really isn't going to improve all that much if you lose weight. If you don't fly because you are too embarrassed to ask for a seatbelt extension, or worse, are afraid you'd be hassled by airline staff, you might "put down" the benefits of taking a vacation with all types of negative predictions about the vacation, from the dangers of flying to sand fleas on the beach and lumpy pillows.

The above ways of thinking exist for a reason. We use them to "protect" ourselves from feeling overwhelmed. They serve a purpose—at least in part. The problem is they are usually short-sighted, outdated habits and cause more harm than good. When looking for your patterns, be cautious about not embarking on a fault-finding expedition, or put yourself down when you discover you have some (or even all) of the above patterns. They are simply ways to help us cope, but in doing so, they may also prevent us from growing and finding better ways of coping. When you discover some less fruitful or even harmful patterns, you're well on your way to trading up for better ways to live and cope. When you discover an undesirable pattern, asking yourself how you benefit from it opens new doors. Always remember to be kind to yourself.

The above process of becoming more aware of your thoughts and how they generate feelings is not just something you set aside a designated time of day to do (although that's not a bad way to get started). Aim to establish a habit of reflecting on your thoughts throughout the day, and especially when you become aware of negative feelings. "Catch yourself" in the act of thinking. Begin to relate your feelings to your thoughts. Do you remember being offered "a penny for your thoughts" when you appeared to be day dreaming? Ask yourself that question frequently. In addition to taking a snapshot of your thinking at any given moment, ask yourself about what you've been thinking the last couple of hours, or what's been on your mind much of the day. The more we "think about our thinking," the faster our progress. This comes with one serious warning: If you are going to be critical of yourself when doing this, don't bother! Do not judge yourself as you discover things. Treat yourself as kindly as you would expect from your best friend. Some people are simply not able to think about their thinking without the guidance of a professional. If that is the case with you, that is perfectly okay. Find a professional to help you.

Hopefully, you will soon be able to identify negative thoughts and biased or distorted thinking. Doing so will help you see your situation more accurately. You'll discover new ways to tackle problems such as overeating. Stand back and look for patterns in your thinking. Patterns do not allow for originality and creativity in thinking.

5. Think Positively

Being aware of your thoughts that lead to negative feelings will allow you to make a conscious effort to change those thoughts to ones that result in more positive emotions. Thoughts are always going to flow, and your internal dialogue is always going to continue. The big breakthrough is when you take command of your thoughts, and replace the negative ones with positive ones. It takes conscious and consistent effort, but the payoffs are fantastic!

Exchange Your Feelings

Once you become aware of your thoughts and how they affect your emotions, you can block certain thoughts and exchange them for more productive thoughts that will result in more positive feelings. Your outcome will be twofold:

1. You can exchange negative thoughts for neutral or positive ones and you will feel better.

2. Becoming more aware of your thinking patterns and distortions will lead to more productive behavior and better problem solving.

Don't think of "banishing" negative thoughts. If you aim to "get that thought out of my head," you've only accomplished half the process. Replace the negative thought with a neutral, or better, positive thought. Here are just a few examples:

A. Replace helplessness with hopefulness.
B. Replace pessimism with optimism.
C. Don't collect injustices. Be forgiving of both yourself and others.
D. Don't focus on yours or other's limitations. Be encouraging to yourself and others.
E. Don't expect bad outcomes. Anticipate positive outcomes instead.

Remember, this is not an exercise like yoga that you practice once a day. Instead, it is a way of interpreting, thinking, and reacting to all the important things in your life; it is ongoing. Change takes time, so be patient. If you make the effort, you will reap the rewards that come from thinking and subsequently feeling differently.

If you find you are unsuccessful in changing your thoughts, emotions, and behaviors, do not think of this outcome as a failure on your part. Instead, it might simply mean you require help to accomplish this. In some cases, it is just too hard to do on your own. Remind yourself that you have plenty of company. Cognitive behavioral therapy can help you make the wanted changes. If you are undergoing a great deal of negative emotion, your best course of action is to work with a cognitive behavioral therapist. The Association for Behavioral and Cognitive Therapies, www.abct.org or (212) 647-1890, can direct you to a cognitive therapist in your area. You can also use self-help workbook such as Christine Padeskey's *Mind over Mood* for depression, or David Burn's *Social Anxiety and Phobia Workbook* for anxiety.

RELAXATION AND OTHER TECHNIQUES

Although preventing the negative emotion from occurring by changing how we think is the best method, we can also calm our emotions through relaxation techniques. The best approach is to use both. Changing how we think and using relaxation techniques is a powerful combination. The basic premise is this: You can't be anxious and relaxed at the same time, and you can teach yourself how to relax. There are a number of techniques you can use. Some approaches to relaxation go back thousands of years to practices such as meditation, mindfulness, and yoga. They all effectively diminish negative emotional states. Biofeedback too can be of assistance in calming one's self.

Meditation, in one form or another, is practiced in most, if not all, of the world's major religions. All the religions seem to have their own unique approaches and objectives. One thing they seem to hold in common is they provide an escape from automatic thinking. Doing so helps us relax mentally and physically (remember that one follows the other). We benefit by focusing our attention on a fixed neutral point rather than allowing our thoughts to wander at the expense of being in the present or having our thoughts provoke feelings. A common component of meditation is to either train or allow the mind to focus on something other than the string of thoughts that usually occur. One analogy is that it is like turning off the engine to let it cool down and rest. Fortunately, many of the same benefits of meditations associated with religious practices can be achieved by non-religious meditation techniques. The non-religious ones are often called "relaxation techniques" or techniques such as "systematic relaxation". Perhaps the most widely one used is "systematic muscle relaxation". All relaxation techniques have a number of benefits:

- Improved blood sugar levels
- Stress reduction
- Muscle relaxation
- Increased immune response (possibly due to less stress)
- Decreased blood pressure
- Improved blood flow to muscles
- Reduced need for oxygen
- Reduction of symptoms such as headaches and back pain
- Better energy
- Better concentration
- Better ability to handle problems

There are many techniques and some specifically ask you to first relax your muscles. Some relaxation techniques skip this and will instead ask y\ou to introduce something to focus on, knowing that once appropriately focused, your body will begin to relax automatically. Below is a general approach that includes meditation. Following this are instructions for systematic muscle relaxation without meditation:

1. Choose a good time of the day to start your relaxation or meditation. Pick two periods of 15 or 20 minutes each, preferably a few hours before bedtime or eating.

2. Find a suitable location away from distractions, especially noise.

3. Get into a comfortable position, which for us is usually sitting. Although sitting up is preferred, you can do this lying down if necessary. One purpose of sitting is to make the body comfortable without inducing sleep. Avoid slouching, dangling your arms, crossing your legs, etc. Keep your feet flat on the floor and your hands resting on your lap.

4. Focus first on your breathing to find a comfortable measured pace. Allow yourself time to relax with your eyes closed. Focus

upon being comfortable and breathe from your diaphragm (belly breathe). Inhale through the nose and exhale out your mouth if possible; however it is not required.

5. Start to relax your muscles by working the muscle groups. This is done by tightening and then relaxing muscles. First start with your toes, then feet, then lower legs, upper legs, stomach, torso, hands, arms, back, and then neck. You can move your neck around a bit very slowly and let it find a comfortable position without dropping forward. Avoid rotating your head to the back. Take time with each muscle group and think of them becoming relaxed, heavy, warm, and finally "dead weight". Eventually, you will learn what relaxation really feels like, and you will be able to do it on command.

6. You now want to focus your mind on something that has a neutral or a positive association but doesn't provoke much thought or reaction. In religious practices, this would often be called a mantra (a repeated word or phrase). So pick a word or very short phrase. Although religious phrases will work, such as "The Lord is my savior," one might be inclined to start thinking about religious beliefs, etc. Try not to contemplate or get into a deep or particular thought; you are trying to do the opposite, to not think, but instead to relax. Good word choices might be: comfort, peace, one, nice, etc. This is the same word or phrase you will use each time. You don't want to change the word because the word or phrase, after it is used repeatedly, will become associated with relaxation and will help you relax more quickly in the future.

7. You will now repeat this word or short phrase silently to yourself in a slow, comfortable manner.

8. As you repeat this phrase, you will find your mind wandering to other thoughts. This is normal and not at all bad; simply bring your mind back to the word or phrase. Do not react negatively to the many times your mind wanders by getting annoyed or upset. To have an automatic thought and not react can actually be beneficial. Simply bring your mind back to the word or phrase the moment you catch yourself "thinking". If something happens to distract you such as a car horn, door slamming, or phone ringing, just accept it without annoyance

and simply bring your mind back to the word or phrase. Life happens and it is okay.

9. If you fall asleep it isn't bad. All it means is that you are relaxed and may require sleep. Bring yourself back to your relaxation exercise and back into the more alert position.

10. Keep a clock or watch available to check the time so you can tell when your 15 or 20 minutes is up. Try to put the timepiece in front of you so you don't have to crane or move your neck to see the time, or grab a pair of glasses. When you check the time, do so slowly and only open one eye and only as far as necessary. Absolutely do not set an alarm! That's like asking someone to slap you when your relaxation period is over!

11. When your time is up, stop focusing on your word or phrase. Remain relaxed for a couple of minutes. Appreciate your relaxed state, and then slowly open your eyes one at a time. Open and close your eyes as often as you like to make the transition gradual. Take your time. When ready, gently start moving one foot, then the other, etc. Make it an easy adjustment from relaxation into your regular state of mind.

12. Let yourself sense your body and how it feels to be relaxed. Enjoy it. Try to take the relaxation with you once your relaxation period is over. You will often realize how relaxed you've become the moment you stand. Be careful when standing because your muscles might be very relaxed and not fully prepared to hold your weight.

13. Get into the habit of making relaxation (or meditation) an important part of every day. The effects are cumulative and the longer you stay with it the more you will get from it. If you can't do it twice a day, which is highly preferable, at least do it once.

In addition to the benefits listed above, if you are becoming anxious or are panicked, you can have a seat, close your eyes, and start using your relaxation (mantra) word. During your daily relaxation routine, your mind has associated the feeling of relaxation to the word you repeat, and you will learn to automatically begin to relax upon silently repeating the word. Being able to meet the fear and anxiety with its opposite, relaxation, is a potent way of dealing with anxiety and anxiety attacks.

Progressive Muscle Relaxation

One of the most popular and effective relaxation approaches, often used by professionals, is called "progressive muscle relaxation". This technique is an exercise in which we systematically tense and then relax the muscles of our body. Doing so teaches us how to relax. It only takes a few minutes a day, and with practice, it very effectively diminishes our FFF response. When we do this, we improve our mood and lower our blood sugar. You can use this as the beginning of the meditation technique described above, or as a stand-alone practice. In either case, practicing it twice a day is recommended. There is an advantage to listening to someone guide you through the technique. There is less pressure on you to remember the next step. You can find many guided relaxation tapes online.

You can also accomplish progressive muscle relaxation on your own. Commit the following to memory so you don't have to stop in the middle of your session to read instructions.

Here are the streamlined instructions:

1. Seat yourself as described in the above meditation exercise.

2. Start by taking some deep breaths, in through your nose and out through your mouth. Throughout the rest of the session, breathing in this manner is recommended. Three or four slow deep breaths will get you off to the right start.

3. If you can (not mandatory by any means), try completing this exercise by using your diaphragm for breathing instead of the secondary breathing muscles in your back and chest. You can determine when you are breathing through your diaphragm by placing your palm on your belly and feeling it go in and out, like a baby's breathing.

4. You are going to tighten your muscles one group at a time. Follow the list of muscle groups identified below. It is important that you do the following with each muscle group:

A. Squeeze and/or tighten the muscle groups listed below, and hold them tight for 3 seconds. Count slowly.
B. Relax the muscle group after the count of three.
C. Feel that muscle group relax, and pay attention to what it feels like for them to relax. Notice the heaviness and warmth.
D. Take another slow and deep breath or two before moving to the next muscle group. Take your time. Hey, this is about relaxing!
E. Move to the next muscle group, and start at "A" above.

5. Here's the order of the muscles groups you will tighten and relax according to the above instructions:

A. Tighten face (both forehead and mouth area) into a ball. Go ahead; use a photo of this on your driver's license if you dare! (Squeeze…)
B. Tighten your neck by tucking your chin into your chest. Do not stretch your neck by twisting it around. (Squeeze…)
C. Tighten your shoulders by bringing them up very tightly. (Squeeze…)
D. Clench your right hand into a fist. (Squeeze…)
E. Extend your right arm and tighten it. (Squeeze…)
F. Clench your left hand into a fist. (Squeeze…)
G. Extend your left arm and tighten it. (Squeeze…)
H. Tighten your stomach muscles. Place your hand on them so you can feel them tense. Don't jump up and wail if you fail to feel six-pack abs. (Squeeze…)
I. Tighten your right thigh. (Squeeze…)
J. Lift and tighten your right leg. (Squeeze…)
K. Tighten your right calf by pointing your toes straight out. (Squeeze…)
L. Curl the toes of your right foot. (Squeeze…)
M. Tighten your left thigh. (Squeeze…)
N. Lift and tighten your left leg. (Squeeze…)
O. Tighten your left calf by pointing your toes straight out. (Squeeze…)
P. Curl the toes of your left foot. (Squeeze…)

6. Once the above is completed, go through each muscle group again in the same order, but this time don't tighten, just take the time to pay attention to how each muscle group feels when relaxed. Nice, isn't it?

7. Relax for a few moments before standing. Stand carefully; your muscles might be too relaxed to immediately support your weight.

EXERCISE FOR RELAXATION

Finally, exercise is an extremely effective way to rid you of a negative emotional state. It improves your mood because it can change a negative mood to a positive one; controls blood sugar levels; expedites weight loss; and most important, it keeps weight off!

We are all very different. The reasons why we overeat and the solutions to our problems are unique for each of us. A lot has been covered, from biochemistry to psychology, but it is meaningless if we can't apply it to our own lives. Perhaps the best way to accomplish this is to apply what we've learned to better understand the lives, struggles, and successes of others. If we come to appreciate their journey, perhaps we can make better sense of our own.

☆   ☆   ☆

Chapter 14

STORIES OF TRIUMPHANT WEIGHT LOSS

The following are accounts of people who have sought help and lost weight. They are based on actual weight loss success stories and problems commonly encountered by people seeking help. They are, nevertheless, fictional. Any resemblance to real people is coincidental.

ALLEN'S STORY: MY WIFE SENT ME

Allen, 41, from Great Britain, has spent the last 10 years living in the US. He is a highly successful owner of a small consulting firm specializing in advertising computer graphics. When given the opportunity, he will tell you he loves his job and is very proud of the business he started from scratch. Upon meeting him, he makes it quickly apparent he is a family man. He is warm, congenial, and appears to be highly intelligent without being stuffy. You can also understand why he is successful in his business: he is very likable, engaging, and comes across as honest. He is living proof that overweight men are not considered "un-smart" as readily as overweight women. He tips the scale at 340 lbs. but is quick to add that much of his bulk is muscle. He is an avid weightlifter. He and his wife of 15 years, Mary, have two children, a boy 12 and a girl 10. He's often referred to as "a regular nice guy". If you meet him, you'll probably agree with this description.

In spite of his weight, he is unusually active. He has a rigorous business schedule, and he is at the gym at least 3 times a week, often four. Weight lifting is his admitted passion. He credits it with helping him relieve stress. His weekday pattern is to start work early in the morning, leave work in mid-afternoon, and stop at the gym for his workout. On those days he doesn't go to the gym. He works late. He also puts in some weekend hours for his business, but usually at home. After his workouts and weightlifting, he stops at his favorite local diner where he often meets up with a couple of friends for a bite to eat and a beer or two. He claims he is "starved" after his workout, and doesn't give much thought to what he eats. His standby, unless something else catches his interest, is a burger and fries. He eats again with his family in the early evening when he is not working late, or later in the evening on those days he works late.

Allen's wife Mary does all the cooking. She enjoys cooking, but he complains, she tends to "ration" his servings because of his weight. He reports he often snacks a few times during the evening, and always has a bite to eat before bedtime. He sometimes washes his snack down with another beer. His wife issues "reminders" critical of his eating throughout the evening. Although he chooses to work with a psychologist/RD, his first interview is conducted by an RD and CDE (registered dietitian and certified diabetes educator).

Session I

Allen gets off to an interesting start. After arriving at the diabetes weight loss center and filling out the forms given him to gather important background information including medical status, he is greeted with a handshake by the intake interviewer, an RD (Registered Dietitian) who is also a CDE (Certified Diabetes Educator). Allen is invited to her office. His wife stands up with Allen and proceeds to accompany him. It is explained politely to her that all sessions are private. Reasons for this are briefly clarified in a warm and reassuring manner. Although her attempt to accompany him is not unusual, her response is: she insists on attending the session with her husband anyway! She protests that if not for her, "He wouldn't even be here!" She scores at least one good point when she says, "His weight affects me as much as it does him!" Oddly, she doesn't sit back down when reassured, but instead remains standing and reiterates, "I will be going in with him." Rather than create a scene in the waiting room, and to prevent others in the waiting room from waging bets on the outcome (it was later reported she was favored two to one), she is invited to the office with her husband to discuss the matter. During these uncomfortable few minutes, Allen is trying to gently coax his wife to accept the rules by reassuring her, "It will be okay honey." When Mary is sufficiently convinced she is not going to be able to stay, she hesitantly agrees to depart for the waiting room. She leaves the office in a friendly manner or, more accurately, makes an attempt to appear friendly and respectful (a pretty good recovery on her part nonetheless)! There's a rumor the waiting room bookie was handing out winnings when she reappeared, but you know how rumors go. You only know the veracity of rumors if you start them yourself.

After Mary's departure from the office, Allen sighs in relief. The RD appears unfazed, but one can only wonder what is going on in her mind. Allen is then asked why he came to the center. His response, a real tension releaser, is "You just met her!" Allen is able to laugh about it, and apparently doesn't make much of the preceding event. He explains he has mixed feelings about coming for help. He knows he is overweight, but is proud that he has been able to prevent his pre-diabetic condition from turning into full diabetes during the last 10 years. He says he is only "a point or two" from falling into the range required for a diagnosis of diabetes. He credits his physical exercise, particularly weight lifting and active life style, for his success. When asked about his weight loss goal, he says he wants to convert some of his weight to muscle. When asked a few more questions, he switches the conversation to discussing options available for losing weight. His father, he is quick to explain, is an important part of his life, and his father lost considerable weight a few years back "the old fashioned way". His father is now strongly advising him to "man up" and attack his excess weight in the same manner he did. Allen stresses it is important for him to please his father, but also says he is curious about lap-band surgery. He admits he knows little about the procedure and his interest in a lap-band is actually his wife Mary's idea. He explains she researched it. He reveals he is secretly not very "keen" on the idea based on the little he's heard.

Allen's goal is general; he says he wants to lose weight and gain muscle. Other than the desire to convert fat to muscle mass, he has a hard time identifying how it would benefit him. He explains he has been overweight since childhood. Being large is part of his identity, and he knows no other way of being. His only other health problem, beyond excess weight, is high blood pressure, which he controls with medication. He admits he has never been asked to think of himself as being average weight. He explains, "As strange as it sounds, I have never thought about it." Although it might sound peculiar to many of us that this highly intelligent man never thought about being average weight, it is actually not that unusual. Some of us apparently believe such goals are so unattainable we don't allow ourselves to fantasize what it would be like. This can work against us because thoughts and visualizations about our desired appearance serve as powerful motivators. In fact, the more specific or detailed they are, the more effective they are! Allen acknowledges that not thinking about weighing less is strange. The question, he admits, gives him something important to think about. He appears amused and intrigued by it as if it is a healthy challenge, not unlike someone daring him to add a few more pounds to his bench press. Allen expects the counselor to repeat everything he has been hearing from his wife: the list of illnesses associated with excess weight, the trauma to his children if he dies early, how it affects his sex life and relationship with his wife, etc. Instead, he shares he is surprised none of the scare tactics are mentioned. Realizing the lack of judgment and absence of lectures, he opens up further: he says he agrees with his father that if he is sufficiently motivated, he could lose weight through willpower alone. But he also admits he has been secretly trying to lose weight, but his attempts have been unsuccessful. He concludes that he must lack sufficient motivation, and admits he is currently not even trying to lose weight. He mock-whispers he hasn't even told his wife about his efforts to lose weight for fear she'd pressure him even more. He makes it clear that he deals better with challenges than he does with pressures. After further discussion, he admits he has a huge appetite, which he calls his "downfall". His worst time, he explains, is after his workouts (but not limited to them he is quick to add). He briefly describes his eating habits. When finished, it appears he might be a binge eater. This is shared with him, along with an explanation of what binge eating means and why it occurs.

He is shocked when he learns during the first session that his ravenous appetite could be related to his blood sugar problems. He protests, "But I don't have diabetes!" As a surprise to him, he receives the following explanation: "It doesn't matter, Allen. Pre-diabetes, like diabetes, can result in blood sugar fluctuations due to diet. This can lead to having an enormous appetite, overeating, and even tiredness." The RD further explains that most pre-diabetics are unaware that extreme cravings and hunger can be the result of blood sugar spikes. Allen is floored. The wheels in his head are spinning. This eloquent, intelligent man is literally speechless, but his grin says it all. When it is suggested he keep a daily food diary in order to gather more specific information about his food intake, he more than willingly agrees. In fact, he appears excited by the project. He realizes he walked into the center with two options: willpower weight loss (which he tried), or lap-band surgery (something he says he really isn't keen on), but is leaving with a third option: being able to address his problem with a change in his diet. Having another option immediately helps him feel more optimistic. He is intrigued by the notion that there might be another way to tackle his problem.

Allen also reveals that he doesn't see an endocrinologist, and his pre-diabetic diagnosis is based exclusively upon HbA1c results. It is explained to him that the HbA1c blood test is a three-month average of blood sugar levels, and there is a chance, based on his report of eating, that the average is a result of both extreme highs and lows in his blood sugar levels. It is recommended that he see an endocrinologist if the result of his next blood test, that just happens to be scheduled in a few days, falls into the diabetic range (126 milligrams of glucose per deciliter or more). He agrees.

He thanks the RD and begins to leave her office. His eyes might even be a little watery; it is hard to tell. There is no doubt, however, that he is very relieved. One can see his body is physically much more relaxed than it was when he first walked in. Part of his reaction, he is later to acknowledge, is because he wasn't judged, and no scare tactics were used. He would agree that belittling is not a valid medical service.

Subsequent Sessions

Mary doesn't accompany Allen to the second session. Surprised? For the second session, Allen meets with a clinical psychologist who is also an RD and CDE. Because of his first visit, Allen is much more relaxed, and feels even more comfortable once he is introduced to the psychologist. Anticipating the psychologist heard of his wife Mary's performance prior to the first interview, Allen makes a joke about his wife's "nagging," and he kiddingly describes how Mary tried to wire him to covertly record their current session. It is clear, after further inquiry, there are no serious problems in his marriage. Allen explains that Mary is now "on-board" because of his positive response to the first session. He is convinced his wife's initial insistence to join the session was out of concern, and he explains she is very protective of everyone in her family. Fortunately, major psychological problems are ruled out during this session. He has the normal ups and downs that most of us have. He noted in his questionnaire he is tired much of the time, but explains it away as probably due to his hectic schedule each day. Three important decisions are made during the second session that lead to the initial steps of putting his support team together.

1. Allen elaborates on his tiredness, and when asked, he describes his sleeping pattern and the problems he is encountering while sleeping. He identifies the following sleep difficulties:

    A. Snoring and gasping at night (as reported mostly by Mary).
    B. Frequent morning and nighttime headaches.
    C. Frequent tossing and turning during the night.
    D. Fear of going to sleep at night. Sleeping, he explains, is far from pleasurable.

Allen also elaborates on his tiredness during the day. Such complaints are common with people who have obstructive sleep apnea, a common problem for people who are significantly overweight. He admits he is usually tired, and that he, "really has to push it". He is convinced his sleepiness is due to his sleep problems and busy schedule—but mostly busy schedule. He adds that he consumes a lot of caffeine to stay wake. With some embarrassment, he reveals he is often afraid to go to sleep. He discloses he often wakes feeling very strange and uncomfortable during the night. He finds this awakening experience hard to describe. He is referred to a pulmonologist to rule out sleep apnea.

Jumping ahead, the pulmonologist recommends a sleep study, and it confirmed he has obstructive sleep apnea. His pulmonologist prescribes a continuous positive airway pressure machine (CPAP) to treat his obstructive sleep apnea. It works by pushing air through a mask or nosepiece that keeps the breathing passages open. It takes Allen a little while to get used to the CPAP machine, and he was tempted to give it up, but within a few days, he is calling it a "blessing". It immediately improves the quality of his life. There is nothing like a good night's sleep, especially when you haven't had one in years!

2. The food diary he has been keeping reveals he is binge eating. When he tries, he finds it easier to control his food intake during the day than he does during the evening. His heaviest eating starts shortly after his workout and continues until he goes to bed. Here's one of Allen's typical days:

TIME	MEAL OR SNACK	Calories
6:00 AM:	Breakfast: Microwavable breakfast sandwich, coffee with cream and sugar	430
7:30 AM:	Pastry and coffee with cream and sugar	250
9:30 AM	Vending machine snack, coffee with cream & sugar	240
12:00 PM	Lunch: Deli sandwich such as corned beef on rye or tuna salad, with chips, and cola	455
3:00 PM	At the gym	0
4:30 PM	Burger and fries. Beer. Sometimes pie, cake, or doughnut, and coffee with cream & sugar	1300
6:15 PM	Cheese and crackers, snack bar, fruit (or anything) and coffee	150
7:30 PM	Dinner: Meat, potato and salad or casserole, salad and beer	750
8:30 PM	Dessert: Cookies, cake, etc.	200
10:00 PM	Cold cut sandwich, beer	550
	Total Calories	**4325**
	Total Carbohydrates	**About 520**

When questioned about eating a sandwich and having a beer before bed, he replies it helps him sleep. It is explained to him that sleepiness and exhaustion often accompany high blood sugar, and the sandwich might be increasing his blood sugar as he heads to bed. It is further explained to Allen that one can become sleepy and exhausted, and even appear to be soundly asleep, but the "sleep" is not restful, because the body devotes its energy to removing the excess blood sugar instead of resting. This, along with sleep apnea, could more than explain his tiredness during the day. Getting his diet under control takes some time. Like many others, he wants help to develop a diet plan that works for him and is satisfying and durable instead of a quick fix.

To help him get his blood sugar under control through diet, he is referred to a registered dietitian counselor who is also a trained chef. Based on his personal food preferences and lifestyle, he and the nutritionist together develop a new eating plan. They both know trial and error are involved in developing a new diet, and keeping a food diary is extremely helpful. Allen agreed at the on-set to keep a food diary. He doesn't make an issue of it. With the prospects of losing weight through an improved diet, especially if the diet can eliminate the extreme "hungers," as he called them, Allen is very enthusiastic. Because he is both a beer and wine drinker, he agrees to switch from beer to a red wine with dinner, and perhaps another one during the evening if it helps him de-crease snacking. Allen's diet successfully reduces his hunger, and because of his success, he can now convince just about anyone of the value of a food diary. If you resist keeping a food diary, he could be persuaded to pay you a "motivational visit", (if you get the drift). He follows the recommended eating plans and recipes, which his wife is happy to prepare, to get his blood sugar under control. Only after gaining some control is he able to build a diet that is suited more to his particular preferences. It doesn't take him much time at all to get to that point.

Allen approaches his new way of eating with a very positive attitude. He knows his diet is a "work in progress," and that en-countering problems with the diet (or his eating behavior) is sim-ply part of the learning curve. Outside of eating to "knock himself out" before bed, he is fortunate in not having many emotional is-sues affecting his eating. In his case, he is overweight primarily because of his particular eating pattern and choices. His old eat-ing style resulted in blood sugar spikes and an extreme appetite.

Allen, incidentally and as part of this diet planning, also has one session with an exercise physiologist. He finds this meeting extremely motivating because of his interest in body building. He learns that it helps to eat a small amount of short-lasting carbs with a little healthy fat and lean protein within an hour before *and* within an hour after his strenuous exercise. This helps his workout and avoids blood sugar surges and dips.

3. To his surprise, Allen finds his next fasting glucose level test falls over the border between pre-diabetes and diabetes. He is technically now a diabetic. As agreed, Allen follows up with an endocrinologist who recommends a glucose tolerance test, a medical test in which glucose is given and blood samples taken to determine the body's effectiveness in clearing the glucose from one's body. The results show his situation is a bit more serious than he thought, even though his HbA1c is just at the normal-high limit. The need for medication is deferred a couple of months with plans to determine the need for medication based upon the success of his new diet and the results of his regular blood sugar testing.

Since refining his diet and dealing with a few obstacles (like most of us, he is not exempt from having a few), he finds he is able to control his diabetes through diet alone, even though he is officially a diabetic. As for Mary, she is doing an extraordinary job learning more about diabetes and the SML diet. In fact, she couldn't be more supportive of Allen, and instead of harping on him because of his snacking during the evening, she joins him in a glass or two of red wine. It is part of their quiet time together. She enjoys the small-, medium-, long-carb recipes, in part because she enjoys cooking and eating a healthy diet. She also reports that her children are more than satisfied with their new diet, possibly because she never makes an issue of it. Allen and Mary are reasonable in their approach and allow their children flexibility, although Mary was a bit more rigid at first than Allen. As a matter of fact, the whole family finds ways to enjoy their favorite foods, as long as they don't go overboard. A year after finishing weekly sessions, Allen continues to manage his diabetes by diet alone. He also continues to use his CPAP, and says his energy is, "through the roof". He is averaging a weight loss of about one pound each week, but frankly, he cares less about pounds than he does his physique. He now gives "healthy eating" the same importance he gives his muscle building. He treats his diet as part of his "wellness package" that includes weightlifting, all of which is part of his lifestyle. He refers many people to the center, but by far, the biggest advocate for the diabetes weight loss center is his wife Mary. She requires occasional reminders, however, not to drag strangers to the center against their will without at least first learning their names.

BRENDA'S STORY: HELP, THEY'RE OUT TO GET ME!

Brenda is the head of the department of communications technology, an undergraduate program in a medium-size suburban college in her state's university system. At 32, Brenda, who has tenure, is safe and secure in her position, but is quick to let you know she feels trapped. "Trapped, poked, and taunted," is her description. She absolutely loves her profession and enjoys keeping up on the latest developments in her field. Her true passion, however, is the classroom. She loves teaching and mentoring her students. They, in turn, find her an exceptionally gifted instructor and caring mentor. She impacts many young lives and refuses to give up her position even though she considers the college a "toxic" work environment.

Her colleagues and the politics that come with her position cause her endless stress. She tells stories of behavior one would never expect to occur in an academic setting. She uses descriptions like "cut throat", and "back stabbing" when referring to her colleagues. The attacks, she claims, are highly personal and more extreme than normal office politics. She is convinced that many of her colleagues are personally out to get her. Although Brenda puts up a strong front and comes across as tough, she is actually very sensitive and easily hurt. She stands up for herself, but she does not retaliate (although she'll admit entertaining a few revenge fantasies from time to time).

Brenda is married, but has no children. She describes her husband, a free-lance graphic artist, as "the perfect mate". He is extremely supportive of her, respects her decisions, and fully supports everything she does.

Brenda's initial paperwork indicates she is 285 lbs. She is seeing an endocrinologist for diabetes, a psychiatrist for anxiety, and an internist for her primary care. She has an unspecified problem with her knees that does not impair her mobility and appears to be related to her weight. Unfortunately, she has hypertension, and it has been getting worse this past year or two. Her most serious medical complaint is that her diabetes is "out of control". Her other blood work results are all within normal limits, including her cholesterol level. Go figure!

Session I

Brenda arrives early for her first appointment and doesn't complain about the numerous forms she is asked to fill out (they are annoying but it is explained they save a lot of interview time). She is greeted by a registered dietitian (RD) and certified diabetes educator (CDE) who introduces himself and invites her to his office. After a few formalities and a moment to settle in, they jump right to the reason for her appointment. When asked what her goal is, she replies with a wide, radiant grin and bright eyes, "To look awesome!" Her reaction lights up the room and the interviewer can't help but share in her enthusiasm with a beaming smile. It is evident that she has her eye on the prize. Little does she know how powerful and important her focus on a goal will be. She'll reap the rewards later. You'll see.

She explains that after toying with the idea of gastric bypass surgery "for years," she is ready to pursue it after being encouraged to do so by her endocrinologist. Her diabetes, she reiterates, is "out of control". She also adds that her psychiatrist encourages her to explore all her options including gastric bypass surgery, and recommends the clinic. Brenda is being treated with medication for anxiety and meets with her psychiatrist monthly. The interviewer recommends she meet with one of the center's clinical psychologists before she is referred to a bariatric surgeon. Brenda is comfortable with this plan, so they set up an appointment with the clinical psychologist.

Session II

Brenda's first session is with the clinical psychologist who happens to also be an RD and CDE (registered dietitian and certified diabetes educator in case you forgot). Brenda and the psychologist cover a lot of ground very quickly, in part because Brenda is immediately comfortable, proves to be an agile thinker, and is an incredibly gifted communicator. She explains she has been heavy since pre-adolescence, and was diagnosed as being diabetic at age 25. She adds that she has been putting on about 10 -15 lbs each year for the last 3 years and is unable to control her weight increase. One of her biggest obstacles, she states, is that she dislikes vegetables (except for the delicious, short-acting, starchy ones we all love). She says she can trace her dislike of vegetables back to her childhood, but believes discussing the origin is "academic" and "unhelpful". She says the same holds true for her history of being abused as a child. She's sure her earlier experiences continue to impact her, but explains she's still left to deal with the consequences regardless of what she's been through. Her admitted downfall is potatoes, in any form, style, or preparation. A review of her usual diet and the results of her blood glucose tests, which she pulls from her handbag, show she is having tremendous blood sugar spikes.

She also explains, without being questioned, that she eats to decrease her anxiety, something she realized long ago. She says her psychiatrist of two years agrees. She tried a weight loss pill some time back, but discontinued it because of the side effects. She makes it clear that her endocrinologist and psychiatrist are on board and supportive of her desire for gastric bypass surgery. The psychologist, based on his interview, concludes that there are no other underlying mental health issues other than the anxiety which she attributes to her work environment. The psychologist finds no reason to not support her desire to pursue the feasibility of gastric bypass surgery, especially because she knows it is only one step of a weight loss process. He will, nevertheless, touch base with her psychiatrist with her permission.

After discussing possible approaches and options, they agree to the following plan:

1. Because they are still dealing with a number of unknown factors, Brenda will continue to meet with the psychologist for weekly sessions for an unspecified period of time. Brenda knows the surgery will have dramatic results, but will not be a total solution. She'll still face the issue of her overeating, especially in regard to decreasing her anxiety. She is comfortable

pursuing a cognitive behavioral approach to changing her eating behavior.

2. Brenda knows the importance of a workable diet. She is open to developing a diet with an RD at a later date—once a decision regarding surgery is made. If surgery occurs, Brenda will require special help to develop a diet plan that is compatible with her gastric bypass.

3. Brenda will be referred to a bariatric surgeon who is part of the center's team for evaluation.

4. Brenda agrees to meet with the program's exercise physiologist to develop an exercise program. Once again, Brenda acknowledges she is fully aware that bypass surgery is only one step in her weight loss program, and she wants a good exercise program regardless of whether or not she gets the bypass.

5. Brenda will continue to see her psychiatrist.

Subsequent Sessions

Brenda, in the opinion of all involved, is a good candidate for gastric bypass surgery. She is unable to adequately control her diabetes through diet and medication alone. This greatly increases her risk of developing diabetes-related health problems. Bypass surgery is performed within six weeks of her first appointment. She finds she is able to control her blood sugar levels almost immediately after her surgery. Consequently, her overwhelming cravings decrease as soon as she gets her blood sugar levels under control. She remains on a diabetes medication. She is also motivated to follow her new, bypass-friendly specialized diet. Like many people, she does best when given specific instructions and detailed diets to follow. It is now 2 years since her surgery. She loses 120 lbs. in the first year, and continues to lose weight slowly, but only, she finds, when she sticks to her new diet and exercises regularly. Also, she has had more than a couple episodes of trying to eat in a manner that undermines her surgery. This is sometimes called, "eating around the bypass". It consists of eating a lot of short-acting carbs so that your insulin level is increased quickly. This increase clears food from the stomach and intestines thereby making room for more food. This undermines the whole purpose of the surgery. Fortunately for Brenda, she learns from her mistakes. Rather than beat herself up, she has colleagues more than willing to do the beating for her.

Brenda continues to see the psychologist on a weekly basis for talk therapy and her psychiatrist for anti-anxiety medication. She still complains of mild anxiety even with the medication, but is learning to use relaxation exercises instead of turning to food to help her relax. She discovers that in addition to using food to lower her anxiety, she is also using it to reward herself; an insight that leads to a dramatic change in her behavior. Further, she comes to realize she is dealing with a tremendous amount of sadness. Food has also provided Brenda some relief from her sadness, and this discovery is just another piece of the emotional eating puzzle. Anxiety, sadness, and reward all contribute to Brenda's overeating, although their influence is greatly diminishing as she changes her thinking.

Brenda is also making substantial progress reducing her anxiety by changing her beliefs about the nature of her workplace and the hidden motivations of the individuals with whom she works. Her situation hasn't changed; it is still brutal. Her perception and reaction to the work-related stress, however, is changing. She is now able to see that many of the conflicts she encounters have more to do with normal politics and her colleagues' dysfunctional coping mechanisms than it does with their intent to do her personal harm. She is making enough progress, and is feeling "awesome" enough, that she is discussing bringing her therapy to a conclusion. She has come to realize that losing weight is not just about what you put in your stomach, but also about what you put in your mind. If you ever were to meet Brenda, you too would agree that she is an "awesome" person. Her students always knew this.

CATHY 'S STORY: SOMETHING IS BETTER THAN NOTHING

Cathy is a 45-year old woman referred to the clinic by her endocrinologist. Cathy has diabetes, and is on a combination of diabetic medications. She weighs 215 lbs., which at 4'8" tall is significant. She is having great difficulty controlling her diabetes.

Cathy reports feeling very depressed. She believes, as does her endocrinologist, that her depression and weight are connected.

Although Cathy is sure they're related, she is confused about how they're linked; she can't distinguish the cart from the horse. She believes she's depressed because she's overweight, and believes she overeats because she's depressed. Beyond that, she finds it all too perplexing and overwhelming. It hasn't even occurred to her that it may be a two-way street, that both possibilities are true. Depression, it's well known, has a way of clouding a person's ability to think clearly. Cathy has yet to realize this even though she's living with it.

Cathy complains of being depleted of energy, and it takes great effort for her just to make it to her appointment at the weight loss and diabetes center. Each day is a struggle just to get to work. She's tried a few diets over the years, but none worked for longer than a couple of months. True to her style, she holds herself responsible for the string of weight loss "failures". It has been a long time since Cathy experienced success in anything in her life, which leads her to conclude that this is as good as life is probably going to get. All but a small glimmer of hope has disappeared.

Cathy is not shy about admitting she is depressed. She declines her primary care physician's repeated offers to prescribe an antidepressant. She's afraid of them and doesn't trust them. She is unsure of what to expect at the weight loss and diabetes center, but at least she's willing to check it out. Her expectations are minimal at best. She feels like she's just going through the paces, walking through a maze that brings you back to where you started.

She is ambivalent about getting help: she simultaneously wants relief from her sadness and depression, and also wants to throw in the towel. She feels unmotivated, extremely sad, unsuccessful, worthless, and hopeless. She also often feels anxious and as if the walls are closing in on her. She has no problem describing her feelings, even though she is not a naturally talkative person. She wants relief from her depression and anxiety, but knows that any solution, if there indeed is one, will also have to address her weight. She definitely feels nervous about her first meeting and musters up all the strength she has to get there on time, which for Cathy is 20 minutes early. Anticipating things will go wrong somewhere along the way to her destination she always gives herself extra time.

Session I

Upon meeting Cathy, the intake interviewer, an RD and CDE, immediately realizes Cathy is depressed or at least very sad. You can see it in her face and posture. When questioned, Cathy describes her home life as "dismal". She says her husband is uncaring and they seldom speak. She explains her son is rebellious and "hangs out with the wrong crowd". She has a job as an administrative assistant in a large company's human resources department, and describes her job as, "better than nothing". She elaborates upon her marriage situation by explaining they have separated a number of times, and are now only living together for convenience. When asked if she ever thinks of divorce and considers looking for a new partner, Cathy laughs for the first time (although somewhat sarcastically) and replies: "Well dear," she says, "I think that train has left the station and there's simply too much baggage remaining on the platform." The interviewer, unprepared for the response, catches herself before she laughs out loud before she realizes how terribly sad Cathy's comment actually is. Cathy smiles a bit, pleased that she is at last able to recall a good line without screwing it up. The interviewer is happy to see a glimmer of wit beneath the sadness. When asked about her support system, Cathy adds she has a few old friends, but is not very active socially outside of "mandatory family affairs". She explains she's usually too tired to go out anyway, and this includes even going to a movie. She adds she hasn't been to a movie in many years. "I hear they have talkies now!" she adds. Without missing a beat, the interviewer replies, "Wait until you see *Gone with the Wind;* it has color and everything!" They enjoy a light moment before returning to their serious conversation.

As an administrative assistant, Cathy does many types of jobs, but mostly record keeping and reference checking. Although she has a fair amount of telephone contact with others, they are usually strangers. She describes her boss as, "power hungry, self-centered, and demanding". She worries she will one day be replaced. She adds that her supervisor, who is in the office next to hers, doesn't seem fond of her. Cathy has been in her position for many years, but her supervisor is relatively new. Cathy is more than familiar with the "out with the old, and in with the new" school of management; after all, she spends a good amount of her time checking references.

The interviewer asks a standard question, "What is your goal? What would you like to be the result of the help you'll receive from our center?" "I'd like to be able to stand on a chair," Cathy replies. Confused, the interviewer inquires, "Why would you want to be able to stand on a chair?" "Well, so my ear can reach the air vent in my office so I can listen in on my boss's conversations!" she responds with a straight face, as if the answer is common sense and obvious. "This way," she explains, "I'll know ahead of time if I'm going to get fired." Because her reason is delivered so sardonically, and not knowing if Cathy is serious or not, the interviewer momentarily freezes…until, that is, Cathy starts to smile. Unfortunately, Cathy finds many days that pass without an opportunity to smile. She's enjoys talking and sharing a small laugh with someone even if it is under these unusual circumstances. Like many of us, humor helps Cathy release some tension.

The interviewer asks Cathy if she's willing to describe what she means by her references to "depression" in the paperwork she completed prior to the interview. Cathy starts to describe how she feels: hopeless, sad, tired, and unmotivated to do much more than eat and sleep. Cathy's eyes become moist as she describes her feelings. When asked if she'd like an appointment with a psychologist, Cathy's ambivalence fades and she replies, with her head down "Yes, please." Knowing an appointment with a psychologist can be intimidating to some people, the interviewer spends the few remaining minutes of the session talking about the psychologist, his sensitivity and kindness. She stresses his success in helping people in her situation and assures Cathy she'll be more comfortable than she probably anticipates. As the interviewer speaks about the psychologist and their center, Cathy begins to perk up. The interviewer describes the results she's personally seen in people in much the same situation as Cathy. She also tells Cathy about all the other specialists on the support team who are available to help her. Cathy begins to make more eye contact and expresses her optimism by repeating "Really?" throughout the conversation. It finally hits home for Cathy when the interviewer explains, "Cathy, this center was built to help people like you." Cathy smiles in relief and asks for the earliest appointment available with the psychologist. As Cathy prepares to depart, she thanks the interviewer by grabbing her hand and says, "I'm looking forward to meeting the psychologist." Cathy finds it unusual to hear herself say, "looking forward" to anything other than a good meal or bed.

The interviewer does not miss the importance of this statement and smiles back at Cathy.

Subsequent Sessions

Cathy greets the psychologist warmly and appears quite comfortable. She opens up immediately when the psychologist asks how he can help her. She describes her current emotional state and problems, and asks for help with her depression and weight. After further discussion and evaluation, the psychologist agrees she is depressed. The option to see a psychiatrist to determine the necessity for an anti-depressant is explored, and although Cathy agrees not to rule it out "permanently," she does not want to move in that direction at this time.

Cathy discusses her home life, and it is clear that she requires help to reduce some of the stress involved in her relationships, specifically with her husband and son. She acknowledges she has very little emotional support, and that her session is, "The first opportunity I've had to talk about myself to anyone in a very long time." She adds, as she breaks into tears, "I have no one to listen to me." Cathy isn't embarrassed by her crying as much as she is disturbed that she is crying when she "should" instead be talking. Cathy is asked about her thoughts while she is crying. One of her greatest strengths is that she is totally open. She seems not to be embarrassed by things that most people often find embarrassing, such as crying, but instead is embarrassed by things she considers violate her strict codes of "shoulds" and "shouldn'ts" she has in her head. Like many of us, she has a lot to sort through. She is reasonable enough to know it will take time. She seems to have one foot firmly planted in the reality of her situation, and another foot bogged down and stuck in a murky world of unreasonable "shoulds" that keep her trapped.

She briefly reviews her past attempts to lose weight, all of which she said she "failed at". It never occurs to her that perhaps the diets failed her. When asked for the finer details of her so-called "failures," it becomes clear that she has a hard time dealing with anything less than perfect adherence to a strict diet. If she "slips up" in some manner even once, she concludes she has blown the diet completely. If she can't hit the bull's eye every time, she considers herself a failure and throws away her bow and arrow. Somewhere during their discussion, she reveals she equates perfectionism with control, and imperfection with lack of control. She wants desperately to have more control over her life, and this only serves to feed her perfectionism. It is also clear that her perfectionism is interfering with her relationships, especially with her son. Moreover, her perfection is boomeranging on her: she expects perfectionism from her son who is bound to fall short of her expectations. The boomerang part is that she considers herself a failure in her role as mother because of her son's lack of perfection. It wouldn't be exaggerating to say that Cathy sets up opportunities to slap herself. She's doing to herself what she later explains was done to her in her childhood.

Related to the expectation of perfectionism is Cathy's tendency to categorize things into "good or bad," "right or wrong," "success or failure," or "black or white". Her greatest challenge is allowing herself the room to be flexible, to be human, to make mistakes and to learn from those mistakes. Learning from your mistakes is a key to losing weight, and it is exceedingly hard to learn from your mistakes when you're preoccupied with beating yourself up. Mistakes, for the most part, are simply miscalculations of expected outcomes. Some of the best discoveries come from mistakes. Cathy requires frequent reminders of this. Many of us do.

It takes a few sessions to develop a plan, and the plan evolves as progress is made. Cathy works on the following:

1. Cathy's food diary becomes a battleground. Being able to keep and use a diary is exceedingly difficult for Cathy. She wants a list of "good" and "bad" foods, and struggles with the importance of allowing some flexibility. For her it is also a question not only of control but of safety—she believes if she's "perfect," she's safer. Cathy has failed to learn from her prior weight loss experiences that given a list of "good" and "bad" foods inevitably results in making an "error," something she can't tolerate making. As soon as she breaks one of her rigid rules, she feels she's failed and gives up. As she starts developing the ability to think about her thinking, she discovers this deep-seated pattern has ruled her life, and that the end result speaks for itself.

She makes a constant effort to keep this "black or white" thinking in check. She's learning a whole new way of thinking. It is not easy.

Cathy meets with a registered dietitian who works on a menu plan with her. Following a plan helps her avoid blood sugar spikes and results in her having a more manageable appetite. In the past, Cathy never had a problem finding a good meal plan; her problem is that she'll scrap the plan if she's unable to stick to it 100 % of the time. If she falls off the proverbial horse, for example, instead of getting back on, her inclination is to beat herself up for being less than a perfect rider even if it is her first attempt at horseback riding. She'd then shoot the horse for good measure so she'll not have to get back on it and risk another "failure". Her problem is allowing herself to be anything less than "perfect". A registered dietitian helps her develop a meal plan that not only includes her favorite foods but is also quick and easy to prepare. This works well for Cathy, because she doesn't like to cook. She commits to keeping a food diary, even if her entries are not 100% according to the plan. It is extremely difficult for her to do this, although she's seeing the benefits of flexibility, and understands the concept of learning from her "mistakes". Old ways of thinking are habitual and take time to change.

2. Cathy continues to see the psychologist and reviews her food diary and reaction to her diet with him. She is able to start dealing with the negative emotions that lead to overeating only after she is comfortable enough to keep an accurate food diary (imperfections and all) and see the connection between her eating and her emotional state. Being able to talk openly about her negative emotions helps her to discover new ways to cope that don't involve food. Cathy also discovers some other thought-feeling patterns that contribute to overeating and depression. It takes a while for her to curtail critical judgments about her thoughts. She is tempted to think of her thinking as "good thoughts" and "bad thoughts". This is unproductive (if not counterproductive), and she works hard to allow subtle shades of gray into her "black and white" thinking.

Once she starts breaking through her depression, which she eventually does, she is less likely to anticipate bad things will happen (this is called "catastrophizing"). In truth, it mostly works the other way around. When she realizes she is having constant thoughts and beliefs that a catastrophe is about to happen, she discovers it contributes to her depression. When she stops herself from anticipating disasters, and replaces the negative thoughts with positive expectations (feeds her brain a healthy diet), it helps her depression to lift.

3. The psychologist teaches Cathy relaxation exercises, and she really takes to them. She practices twice a day…religiously! It helps her anxiety, which along with reducing her "catastrophizing," helps her reduce her overall anxiety.

4. Cathy meets with an exercise physiologist and starts an exercise program. She starts walking regularly, and wears an accelerometer that monitors her physical activity and calories burned each day. It is an armband or wristwatch-like device, and it fits on top or under her clothing.

5. Cathy makes a sincere attempt to work on her relationship with her son. Simply having the opportunity to talk to the psychologist about their relationship, and helping her develop the "think about your thinking" skills improves her relationships. She also has the goal to increase her social life beyond "family obligations". Her exercise physiologist recommends she find a physical activity that is fun. She would like to start dancing, she reports.

6. Cathy starts to search for enjoyable pastimes and activities that add satisfaction and a sense of mastery to her life. She has discovered dancing and she is a bit more social, but has a hard time finding ways to have fun.

Update:

It has been two years since Cathy started working with the center's team on weight loss. She continues to see the psychologist weekly, and much of their work centers on changing the thoughts related to her depression and overeating. They also spend time working on forming more satisfying relationships. She never decides to give antidepressants a try. Although she understands the explanation that treatment isn't a choice of *either* medication *or* talk therapy, and that she can have both, she is unconvinced. Nevertheless, the quality of her life has improved greatly, and she is definitely much less depressed. Her overall improvement is apparent to everyone who knows her. Now, sit down for this one: She has lost 80 lbs. during the two years and now weights 135 lbs.! She feels good, looks good, and has taken up dancing in addition to her impressive 10,000 steps a day (this equals 5 miles) routine as measured by her accelerometer (which she refers to as her boyfriend, because it is her constant companion)! The thinking patterns that worked against her and were part of her depression remain in a "much weakened state". As she slowly reveals more information about her childhood, it is easy to appreciate why she developed the thinking patterns she did. In final analysis, and considering what she endured in the past, she is a tremendously strong and resilient individual to be overcoming as much as she is.

Cathy still has some very hard times, however. There is hardly a week that goes by that doesn't bring new challenges. Like most of us, she slips back into some of her old patterns when stress is high. She hit bottom when she was fired before losing enough weight to stand on the chair to listen to her boss's plan to "can" her. It took her a long time to find a new job, and it was a particularly difficult time for her. She now says, "If I made it through that, I can make it through anything." She has a new job and her new boss reminds her much of her old one. The exception is her new boss hired rather than inherited her. She's on the "in with the new" team now. Her office is a cubicle, much better for eavesdropping, but her boss is safely behind sound-proof walls.

As part of creating her new lifestyle, Cathy started expressing interest in developing a better relationship with her husband, and discussed her marriage in therapy. Although she hasn't succeeded in getting him to attend marriage counseling with her…yet…she no longer refers to him as "the sofa that occasionally moves and pays rent". To her surprise, he has shown interest in her personal growth and joins her in her SML meals. For the first time in years, usually over meals, they are actually talking about their relationship. Cathy discovered that she had a pattern of painting herself into corners because of her rigid "rules". Her "rules" had all the flexibility and warmth of governmental laws. As her rigidity decreased, her relationships improved, especially her relationship with her husband.

As for her son, he is 17 and eats whatever is in front of him. He is changing so fast that it is impossible to discern if progress in their relationship has been made or not. She reports he's a loving son, a rebellious kid, disrespectful brat, hormone-driven teenager, a child, a young man with great promise, and a handful. Oh, she goes to the movies once in a while now, and absolutely loved *Gone with the Wind*!

Chapter 15

CHOOSE HAPPINESS AND FIND SUCCESS

We are obviously all different, and each of us will have a different experience losing weight and managing our diabetes. Some of us simply want a food eating plan that helps us control our hunger and we'll start to lose weight. Allen, our weightlifter, is a good example of this type of person. All he has to do is stick to an SML eating plan and the rewards are almost automatically bestowed upon him. People like Allen don't have to concern themselves with issues of emotional eating; he'll lose weight, build muscles, and have a less critical wife almost automatically. For Allen and all of us, losing weight alone has many benefits. Remember, benefits function as our rewards and include:

- A sense of personal accomplishment
- Increased self-esteem
- Increased self-confidence
- Strong sense of empowerment
- Complements from others
- Being treated better by others
- Improved health
- Increased physical stamina
- A wider range of physical activities in which we can comfortably engage
- Feeling less self-conscious
- Greater physical comfort
- Decreased health lectures from people, etc.
- A fabulous example for others

Whereas it appears the above list provides substantial enough rewards to lose weight, some of us, particularly those of us who eat at least in part for emotional or psychological reasons, may have to increase our rewards. We've already discovered that *The Greenwich Diet* isn't only about eating SML meals and feeding ourselves positive thoughts, it is also about finding ways to reward ourselves. We want to "sweeten the pot". By sweetening the pot, we're tipping the balance in our favor. To tip the balance in favor of our success, we'll want to discover new ways to live that rely less on food to help us sustain our emotional needs. Because we'll still want the satisfaction we once got from food, we'll want to look for satisfaction elsewhere, because the desire for satisfaction doesn't go away just because we lose weight. We're therefore all off on our own personal treasure hunt to:

Find new sources of pleasure we once got from food.

Discover new ways to decrease our anxiety when we're anxious.

Find new ways to reward ourselves and to celebrate that it doesn't involve (too much) food.

The Importance of Food

Don't underestimate the importance of food in your life. Respect the fact that it provides pleasure and helps you maintain emotional balance. It is also an incredibly effective reward! You don't overeat because you are bad, weak, greedy, selfish, out of control, an animal, or any other offensive term you've heard or thought. You eat to take care of your feelings (in addition to responding to some wild bio-chemical demands you've already learned about).

Unfortunately, unless you are similar to Allen, your emotional needs won't automatically disappear with a change of diet. That's not how it works. Darn. If food is your reward system, a way to celebrate, a quick way to calm down, or an immediate pick-me-up, you'll want to find those supports elsewhere. Don't make the mistake of thinking you can do without them; you'll only be able to ignore them for a short while, or you'll become wonderfully thin and exceedingly unhappy.

If you are one of the many of us who eats to balance your emotions, you'll find that being able to satisfy your emotional needs elsewhere is an essential part of a permanent weight loss solution. You'll want to do some serious thinking and rearrange your life to insure you get your rewards and emotional satisfaction from things other than food. This rearrangement of our lives takes, at times, as much effort as sticking to our SML approach to eating. To successfully lose weight, and maintain our weight loss, not to mention being happy, we'll want to change our life around. For lack of a better expression, let's refer to this transformation as a "lifestyle change".

Motivation and Goals

The rewards that come with weight loss are our motivators. Motivation is what gives us the strength to avoid overeating, gets us to exercise, encourages us to practice our relaxation exercise, etc. Achieving our long-term goals is our ultimate reward, but we also might want to have many smaller goals to reward us for our progress along the way. It's not unlike celebrating every single pound we lose, but it's much better because we don't have to use a temperamental scale. Just knowing we are making progress toward our goals is motivating, and nothing breeds success like success! Our goals will come to our rescue when we remind ourselves of their importance as we talk our way around the temptation to overeat from the conveyor belt of tempting foods that passes before us each day. Because goals are so vital to our success, what we choose as goals and rewards are extremely important.

Stay Positive

We've learned from experience that denying our desires and torturing ourselves into losing weight is not a viable long-term solution. It leads to unhappiness, short tempers, lousy dispositions, fewer invites, and cheaper holiday gifts. We don't want punishments (especially self-imposed ones). We want rewards. We much prefer carrots to whips, and fortunately, carrots are more effective. If we can learn how to redirect our appetite for food into an appetite for living, enjoyment, and long-term satisfaction, we can transform our lives. If you make this transformation from short-term thinking and quick gratification mood stabilizers to long-term focused living, the payoffs, once achieved, last much longer. If you can develop an SML diet that provides you an acceptable level of satisfaction, you are again helping tip the balance in the desired direction. You can also tip the balance further in your favor by having clear, personally meaningful goals. Fantasize about the rewards that will come to you when you lose weight: the pride you see in your own eyes when you look into the mirror; the ability to move more freely; your attractiveness and sexiness; and how you'll be perceived differently. Think beyond the standard list of payoffs and personalize them. Use your imagination; fanaticize and visualize what lies ahead for you. Remind yourself of your personal goals often, think about your thinking, and remember you "want" food, you don't "need" it (except in extreme cases). If you do this, you can create both a thinner and happier life.

Think Clearly About Your Goals

Some benefits come directly to us simply because we lose weight, but when we talk about lifestyle change, we may want to expand our way of thinking about goals. Often, our goals are not one grand step, but require a few smaller steps before we reach them. For example, if you're in a bad relationship and appease your sorrow with chocolates, and you have the goal of finding that "special someone," you may have to bring one relationship to an end; recover emotionally; find new friends and social activities; brush up on your dating skills; whiten your teeth; shop for new clothes; explore local dating opportunities; check out social networking and Internet dating sites, etc. This is breaking the ultimate goal down into smaller, incremental steps. Reaching each small step feels fantastic! You'll experience tremendous satisfaction each time you achieve every one of the smaller goals leading up to the jackpot. Sure, it's okay to measure your success in pounds, but it also pays to measure your success in other ways that truly matter to you. Keep your ultimate personal payoffs and the life you want to create for yourself foremost in your mind. Your goals are extremely important. *Not only do they keep you motivated, the pleasure and satisfaction they provide can replace some of the pleasure and satisfaction you once got from eating!*

Find "Start Here" on Your Map

To set some great goals, you'll want to be mindful of what thoughts are related to your emotional eating. Some of us see the connection immediately and clearly. Others of us don't, even the most astute of us. The key, of course, is learning to think about your thinking, and to do so without being critical. Being noncritical is often the hardest part for many of us. Some of us might want help to figure out our food-emotion connection because it is not always a clear connection. More than a few of us could benefit from professional help. Some of us might want to get professional help just to check to be sure we're on the right track (no one can see their blind spots or they wouldn't be called blind spots), and others of us simply want to take an express train toward our goals. Professional help offers the opportunity to explore our innermost personal thoughts in a safe, non-judgmental setting. Seeking help as a first step is a smart move for many, but others of us might want to attempt to understand our emotional eating on our own. You can always seek help later if you find you are not making progress. A large number of us can and will successfully tackle our emotional eating problem on our own. Like target practice, it might take time to hit the bull's eye, so be patient, learn what works (and doesn't), and most of all, don't become critical or discouraging of your efforts. As an important reminder, the task is much easier if you first get your blood sugar levels under control and pay close attention to the wild biochemistry involved in hunger and eating. Trying to tackle the emotional component of overeating while you are on a blood sugar rollercoaster is going to be very frustrating if not impossible.

Goals Change as We Change

Our goals may change over time as we live, learn, adjust to life, and lose weight. Give yourself a green light to change your goals when and as you see fit; after all it is your life and your goals. Once you are close to achieving your goal, things may feel or look very differently. You might want to have small goals, medium goals, and grand goals—as many or as few as you want and in any combination you want. They can be highly ambitious, modest, or a combination. As long as they are true to who you are and motivate you, and they come from the long-term thinking part of your brain, they're all good. If you keep your super long-term, ultimate, extravaganza goal of having an enjoyable life in mind, any goal that helps you get there (as long as it is legal!) is a good goal.

Maintenance and Sliding Back

To err is to be human. If you waver from your new lifestyle, brush yourself off and try to find the reason why it happened. Don't fall into the trap of self-blame! Ask yourself: do you want to modify your diet, set new goals, remind yourself of them more often, build in more incentives, or is the waver emotionally based? Keep an open mind, stand back, and evaluate what's working and what's not working for you in the new lifestyle you are developing. Hey, your life is always a work in progress! Make the changes you want to make, and if you don't find anything to fix or change, don't dwell on it. Just say "oops," brush yourself off, and jump back on the horse. Focus on the ride, not the fall. Don't be like Brenda and beat yourself up, and for goodness sakes, don't shoot the horse!

Add Value to Your Life

As you think about long-term goals that help offset the emotional things you get from food, think about setting goals as future opportunities to be able to engage in behaviors and activities that add the most value to your life. The more you value something, the more you'll be motivated to get it. If you engage in things you truly value (be they conventional or not), you'll feel proud of yourself and be happy—the ultimate payoff. People who live their lives according to their personal values are happier than those who don't. If you engage in things that do not reflect your personal values, you'll lack joy. It is that simple.

So how do you set goals that maximize the rewards? To start, your goals have to be in line with those things you value the most. The things you value most in life are called "life goals," "personal values," "cardinal virtues,"or "core values". They all mean much the same thing, and they are the things in life that mean most to you, things you value the most. They define much of who you are, and they are your compass in life. Here's just a short list of some personal values to help you get the idea:

- Kindness
- Independence
- Raising a family
- Justice
- Helping others
- Honoring commitments
- Achievement
- Having fun
- Good health
- Physical appearance

- Strength
- Valor
- Wealth

It is often said you can't reach your goal if your "heart" isn't into it. We often talk about things we value and our passions as if they "come from the heart". Love, passion, commitment, desire, value, and indeed all awareness and thought, however, come from our brain not our heart. Our heart simply pumps blood. It has no awareness. It has no passion. Sure, our heart react to our thoughts (as well as other stimuli) by speeding up or slowing down, but it doesn't have feelings. "You gotta have heart" is really "You Gotta Have Awareness". Nevertheless, if an idea gets you excited (other than one arousing fear or anxiety of course) and your heart pump a bit faster to prepare for action, you're probably onto something powerful! Get excited, but don't wait for your heart to arouse your passion. Let your passion arouses your heart.

Many of us don't stop to think about or identify our core values any more often than we stop to contemplate electricity, yet both core goals and electricity are invisible forces that supply energy. If you want help identifying your core values, think about the person you are and how you would like to be in the major areas of your life, such as: career, family, physical appearance, health, religious or spiritual life, relation-ships, special interests and hobbies, fun and entertainment, etc. If you live life in accordance with your core values, you'll be happier. When it comes to goal setting, the more your goals reflect and express your core values, the more powerful they will be. The more powerful they are, the more motivated you will be to achieve those goals, including goals related to your weight loss and new lifestyle. Adding as much detail to the goals as you can also helps. Developing goals that bring your core values to life is the secret of motivation.

Although core values eventually lead to behavior, there are a few very important steps in between. You'll recognize some of the steps from earlier discussions:

Core Values
The things you believe are most important in your life.

Beliefs
Things you believe because of your core values. This is sometimes
called your "belief system".

Rules for Living
If you have values and beliefs, you have to have some rules to help
guide you to live up to your values and beliefs.

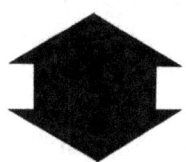

Automatic Thoughts
Automatic thoughts are the constant dialogue, feedback, conversation or mind-chatter in which you engage. The thoughts can be your
way of constantly evaluating, reminding, scaring, worrying, soothing
yourself, or habitual ways of keeping your mind occupied.

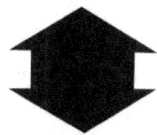

Feelings

Feelings are emotional reactions to things, real or imagined, happening in our world, including our own thoughts and interpretation of events. Feelings usually have labels such as "happy," "sad," "regretful," "frightened," etc. Feelings are both a mental awareness as well as a corresponding physical response in our body.

Behavior

Behavior refers to all of our actions, from putting on our shoes in the morning, smiling at our children as we send them off to school, to breaking into a pastry shop dressed in a clown's outfit.

Once you identify your core values, give thought to your beliefs and the rules you've created to support your core beliefs. You can identify your beliefs and rules by thinking about your thinking (mindfulness). Awareness of your thoughts is of paramount importance to change your eating behavior. If you eat (a behavior) for emotional reasons (feelings), remember that feelings are based on thoughts. Many of those thoughts are automatic. To change your eating behavior, you'll want to become aware of the thoughts that generate the feelings, and then change your thoughts. It requires repetition—much repetition. Through repetition, we can change automatic thoughts. If you change your thoughts, you can change your behavior. This is the crux of cognitive behavioral therapy. Changing your thoughts takes time, so be patient with yourself. You cannot change automatic thoughts overnight. They've been popping into your head for years, but if you stick with catching and changing those thoughts to more positive and realistic ones, your brain will eventually change. Positive thoughts will eventually automatically pop into your head.

Although thoughts generate feelings, many of us are all but oblivious to our thoughts but highly attuned to our feelings. For us, the key is to monitor our feelings, and when we realize we're experiencing negative feelings, immediately identify the thoughts that are going along with these feelings. If you do this, you'll start to see patterns in your thinking and feelings. You can change the thought, but remember that feelings are "sticky" and will remain around longer than you would like. Do not expect to see instant results. Keep at it, however, and you'll get results!

The above "Core Goals" diagram is useful in two ways:

1. You can start at the top of the chart and increase your motivation to lose weight by developing goals that are based on your personal core values. Think from the top down (core values to behavior) and set goals that enhance your chances of being successful.

2. Using the chart from the bottom to the top helps you trace your behavior upward into thoughts, rules, beliefs, and values. You might notice a problem at any point. What are the thoughts, rules, beliefs, or values that lead to overeating? Although overeating might give you a little boost, it is not going to lead to a more satisfying life.

Confused and a little overwhelmed by the above? Tempted to come to the conclusion this is a bit too deep, and you'd prefer just to move on? Don't give up yet. Let's look at how the above fits a few people you know: Allen, Brenda, and Cathy.

Allen

Allen has some very clear *core values*. He defines himself as a family man and everyone who knows him agrees he lives up to his *values*. His life and behavior reflect these *values*. He *values* his body, specifically his masculinity and muscles, and his behavior (working out at the gym) reflects this *core value*. He *believes* you have to stick to things to accomplish them. He even plugged his SML eating plan right into his *value* of desiring a muscular body. His new diet is almost effortless because it is aligned with his *core value* (a supportive wife who does all the cooking doesn't hurt either!) and after each meal he *feels* good that he is sticking to his new diet. He *values* his independence and built a career that allows him this. His self-made business adds greatly to his overall *feelings* of happiness in life. He is not particularly religious, but he has a strong moral code (moral *core value*) and it is reflected in his friendships and his business practices. It is a great part of his reputation and success. He enjoys spending time relaxing at home with his wife, and adding a bottle of wine to the evening was also right in line with this *core value*. Allen's moral character, a *core value*, is also the basis of the *rules* by which he lives, fidelity, being honest in his business practices, not lying, not breaking promises, etc. All of these *rules* he created by which to live are based on his personal *belief* system that says, "What you cast out comes back to you". As for his *automatic thoughts*, he is a good example of how effective and powerful *positive* automatic thoughts can be. When working, he is constantly saying things to himself like: "Wow, you aced that one!" "I'm just keeping it honest!" "They know they can trust me!" "I sure am good at what I do!" etc. Consequently, he *feels* great most of the day. In the gym, he reminds himself of how good he looks and what a hard worker he is. When he walks in the door at night, he reminds himself of what a wonderful family he has, and what a good father he is. He *feels* great that he's a success in his own eyes. Frankly, Allen's weight loss was rather easy. This is because he has few emotional issues to work through and his life is an expression of his *core values*. We should all be so lucky!

Brenda

Remember Brenda, our technology professor who had gastric bypass surgery? She works as a department head in a local college and *believes* she is "harassed" by peers who are personally out to get her. She has some very clear and strong *core values* as reflected in her lifestyle. She states her goal is to look "awesome". A good physical appearance is obviously important to Brenda, but she *believes* she hasn't lived up to her expectations for many years prior to her surgery. She *feels* bad about this, guilty, and has to change those thoughts when they enter her mind. She has strong *core values* especially concerning education and professionalism, and she has an exceptionally strong work ethic that is reflected in her *beliefs* and *rules*. Her *core values* lead her to *believe* you have to work hard to get ahead. She also *believes* it is a very competitive world out there, sometimes cutthroat.

These *beliefs* are evident in her choice of career, preparation for her career, keeping up to date on advances in her field, and her love of the classroom. She *feels* what she calls a "high" right after class. As a matter of fact, keeping up to date on things and meeting her many obligations are some of the *rules* by which she lives. Her *rules*, as they are for all of us, are based on her *beliefs*. Although she denies being religious or spiritual, she brings a special fervor to her mission to educate young adults and zeal to helping them develop personally and professionally. In many ways, she is passing on her *values, beliefs,* and *rules* to the next generation—or at least trying. In this respect, her mentoring seems to fulfill her desire to nurture. She's in a strong, committed relationship. She is bold and brave, exemplified in both her decision to have gastric bypass surgery and her willingness to put up with a hostile work environment in order to continue in her position. Simply put, she has a *core value* to work hard, *believes* hard work pays off, establishes *rules* such as "don't go to bed until the exams are graded," "work even when you're sick," "if you are going to do something do it right the first time," etc. Those *rules* make themselves known in her *automatic thoughts*. Those thoughts result in *feelings*, and her *feelings* lead to her *behavior*. Although she is true to her *core values*, and even her *beliefs* are aligned, her *rules* don't leave much wiggle room. If she doesn't have wiggle room, it is unlikely that she allows others to have wiggle room either. This might explain some of her reaction to her peers, or their reaction to her.

Her strong work ethic and desire to excel has led her to *believe* that her strengths are being used against her by those who don't share her *values*. She sees her peers as being rather lazy, far too political, and she *believes* they want her "done in". She *believes* their undermining and uncooperative behavior is personally directed at her, and ulterior motives are at play. She also *believes* that only the strong survive, and she is therefore willing to endure the hostile environment.

Brenda's *core values* of being strong support her *belief* that it is important to forge ahead. She establishes *rules* such as "don't waste time". This, in part, is why she is so "head strong". She understands that bypass is not a one-step solution. She participates fully in everything recommended after her surgery. It's like she is on automatic pilot because of automatic thoughts (for example, "just do it").

As you see, Brenda has many *rules* for herself *and* others. Her *rules* center on expecting maximum performance from herself and everyone, keeping your nose to the grindstone, overcoming obstacles, and setting high expectations. In fact, she can rattle off many *rules* to support her *beliefs*. She thinks of her *rules* as her guidance system, her internal GPS. Sometimes, our greatest strengths also become our greatest obstacles, but that's for Brenda to decide; after all, it is her life.

Many if not most of Brenda's *automatic thoughts* are in compliance with her *rules*. The downside to her many rules is she is constantly evaluating her performance, setting high expectations and not giving herself much of a break. This feeds her depression, and provokes dissatisfaction with others who she perceives as "lackadaisical" or "lazy". Her high demands of herself, and fear of not living up to her own high standards, create anxiety for her. Eating calms her down, elates her, and temporarily turns off the *automatic thoughts* that are constantly providing feedback and self-evaluations.

Brenda lives in an almost constant state of anxiety because of her work situation, and her *belief* that her peers are personally out to get her, something she later acknowledges is a distortion. She eventually comes to see that her peers' behavior toward her is not as personal as she once thought. She begins to notice how they treat each other, and also comes to appreciate that each of her peers has his or her own struggles, limitations, and yes, dysfunctional ways of coping. Brenda, like many of us, wants to "tweak" some of her *beliefs* so they fit reality a bit better. She *feels* less threatened when she starts decreasing the automatic thoughts that have been telling her to watch her back. The *automatic thoughts* came from her *rule* that you always have to be diligent around peers. You can trace her feelings all the way up to her beliefs, and even see how they are based on her core values.

Over time, Brenda comes to see that her *rules* are often too rigid, and her *automatic thoughts* are more harassing than her peers' behavior toward her. Her constant *automatic thoughts* that persistently evaluate her own performance, such as, "You can do better than that!" have been replaced with, "Another great job girl!"

Although she still struggles with some depression and anxiety, in part because of her rigid approach to life, her weight loss goals are fully supported by her *core value* system, and are almost effortless. Consequently, she had no problem adhering to her new lifestyle, and thinks she's "awesome".

Cathy

Cathy was very depressed when she sought treatment. It is much harder to define Cathy's *core values* than it is Brenda's. At best, one could say they are centered around being stoic, accepting things for the way they are, maintaining a sense of humor. Actually, Cathy has a very hard time identifying her *core values*. At times it seems like she is even fighting against them. She has been bogged down in *beliefs* and *rules*, many of which are unrealistic and usually rather harsh and unforgiving. Sometimes people *feel* there is something so pervasively wrong with them that *believe* they seem unsalvageable or even "rotten to the core". This is the case with Cathy. She truly believes she is fundamentally flawed. This mistaken *"core value"* leads to *beliefs*, *rules*, and *automatic thoughts* that are rigid, cruel, and ultimately lead to depression. She *values* family but gave up on having a perfect family—except, perhaps, expectations concerning her son. She doesn't *value* work, she has to work. She'd much prefer to be a homemaker. Cathy is more in survival mode than living a fulfilling life. Many of us are in her shoes.

Cathy holds herself responsible for her failures: a bad marriage, a low paying job, a rebellious son, her weight, lack of an adequate social life, etc. Her self-criticisms are due, in part, to her *belief system* that says you are responsible for your own destiny. Her *automatic thoughts* constantly badger her and remind her of her failures. She seldom notices her accomplishments, and credits her few successes to "following the *rules*". She settles for simply wanting to exist with the least pain possible. Just about anything is "better than nothing," as she often says. In fact, the problem is that she is trying to live a *value system* that is not of her own creation. It was drilled into her as a child or perhaps is just a child's reaction to poorly-equipped parents. Her *core values* are someone else's *core value system*. It takes Cathy time to identify her personal *values* and develop a new *value system* that is authentically hers. Cathy is far from alone. Many of us spend our lives trying to live up to someone else's *value system* (often parents) or expectations. We try to please others instead of ourselves.

Until Cathy finds her own way, she is just following a script created for her by someone else. Unfortunately, she is like an unprepared actress who stumbles onto the wrong set. She is constantly falling short of her own expectations; and she is constantly putting herself down through *automatic thoughts*.

Because she is walking an emotional tightrope and *believes* grave consequences will follow if she doesn't keep perfect balance, she *believes* everything has to be perfect or she'd fall or fail. She lives in a world of "shoulds and shouldn'ts," "rights and wrongs," "good thoughts and bad thoughts". These are all *rules* based on her *beliefs*. She has to first look at her *behavior*, and then connect the dots to her *automatic thinking*. Only then can she take the leap of examining the *rules* and *beliefs* behind them. In other words, some of us benefit from working from the bottom of the diagram up, questioning the validity and consequences of our *thoughts, rules,* and *beliefs* that result in our *feelings* until we find the part in the chain that is not working for us. Cathy is realizing that living our lives in accordance to *values* we inherited, unknowingly adopted, or *values* that were imposed on us, don't often lead to happiness. As she discovers who she really is, Cathy would suggest we all could benefit from stopping to examine our *core values*, and insuring that the *values* we live by are genuinely ours. We have the right to be authentic and true to ourselves.

Value Based Living: Life According to Your Values

Like Cathy, much of life seems to just "happen" to many of us, leaving us trying to cope with the present, hold our wits together, and adjust to changes. The idea of "planning ahead and designing our lives" seems quite lofty to some of us. More than a few of us have given up trying to set personally satisfying goals; we're just treading water and seeking basic security. Some of us have been disappointed and burnt so many times when it comes to setting personal goals, we've given up thinking about them altogether. We feel goal setting is just another set up for disappointment. Don't give into the PPP (poor pleasure prediction), not at this time, regardless of your track record of disappointments. Some of us didn't have the opportunity to get off to a good start in life, and certainly many of us lacked opportunities or faced great misfortunes over which we had little or no control. Some of us currently struggle with being able to afford even basic necessities like a roof over our heads or putting food of any type on our table. Yet, regardless of where you are now or where you've been and how you feel, now is the perfect opportunity to stand back, take a compassionate look at your life, think about what is really important to *you* and decide to live the rest of *your* life according to *your* personal values to your best ability.

If you engage in activities you truly value, you will be happy. Think back to when you felt extremely happy. Was it when you lost a significant amount of weight in the past? Was it when you were married? Single? Was it when you received a job offer, promotion, or raise? Was it when you joined a group, received a compliment, or did charitable work? Doing things you value brings happiness. The problem is that many of us say we value things but, in truth, we may be using another person's values, or something we were told we "should" value. Think about it. Think about yourself and what brings you happiness. Think about your thinking. Also, think about this:

1. What two activities take up most of your time?

2. How do you feel about yourself after you're done with those activities? Do you feel good about yourself or happier?

So, how do you stand far enough back to take a compassionate look at the whole of your life? Think about the end of your life, of course! When you pass from this earth, how do you want to be remembered? How do you want your epitaph or tombstone to read?

Here lies someone known as Kate,
Who always worried about what she ate.
She only valued her health and weight,
So don't let her obsession become your fate!

Or

Here lies a loved one we call Kate,
The perfect friend, a loving mate.
She didn't leave a large estate,
But what a life she did create!

This book started on a very personal note, so it is fitting that it ends on one. Your weight loss journey will be different than mine. We're all different. I lucked out because my journey included a chance meeting with my co-author Chris. I met Chris because I live only 7 minutes from where he practices. Chris, the kind of professional who doesn't plaster his wall with his degrees, had no problem with the idea of turning his professional work into a self-help book—a proposal that would have offended some experts. He simply wanted to help people by getting the word out. He has a passion for his work.

I wouldn't say my weight loss (thus far) has been easy, but it sure was easier than I anticipated. I certainly got more out of it than I put into it. I also came to value the support of others, especially professionals. Asking for help isn't a sign of weakness; it is a sign of commitment, strength, and optimism. That's why the first step is the hardest and most important.

I slowly created a new lifestyle that's much better than my old one. Although I initially aimed for the light at the end of the tunnel (measured in pounds), I found the tunnel had many lights along the way. I came to realize that enjoying life was the big goal I was always after, and losing weight was just a means toward an end. I can no longer separate the quality of my life from my weight loss—they are a package deal. To my surprise, I have no fear of sliding back either. I can live with my new lifestyle and my new way of eating. That blows my mind even more than the number of pounds I've lost. I'm probably the type of person who will have to keep a food diary the rest of my life, but frankly, it's no big deal. It is a small price to pay.

Thank you Chris for your willingness to share your knowledge with others, and for the help you've given me.

On behalf of Chris, the many others who contributed to this book, and me, may you find yourself becoming thinner, healthier, more satisfied, and happier.

✷   ✷   ✷

End